JOSETTE MILGRAM

MAKE UP

marie claire

MURDOCH BOOKS

make Up

maquillage
[makijaz]
ふんしょく
trucco
maquillaje
urechtmachen
化妝
kosmetika

Contents

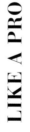

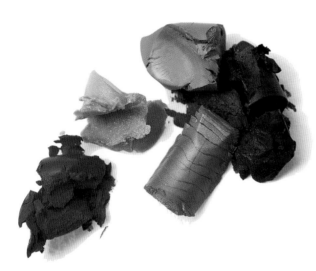

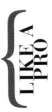

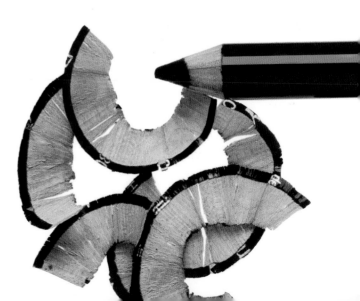

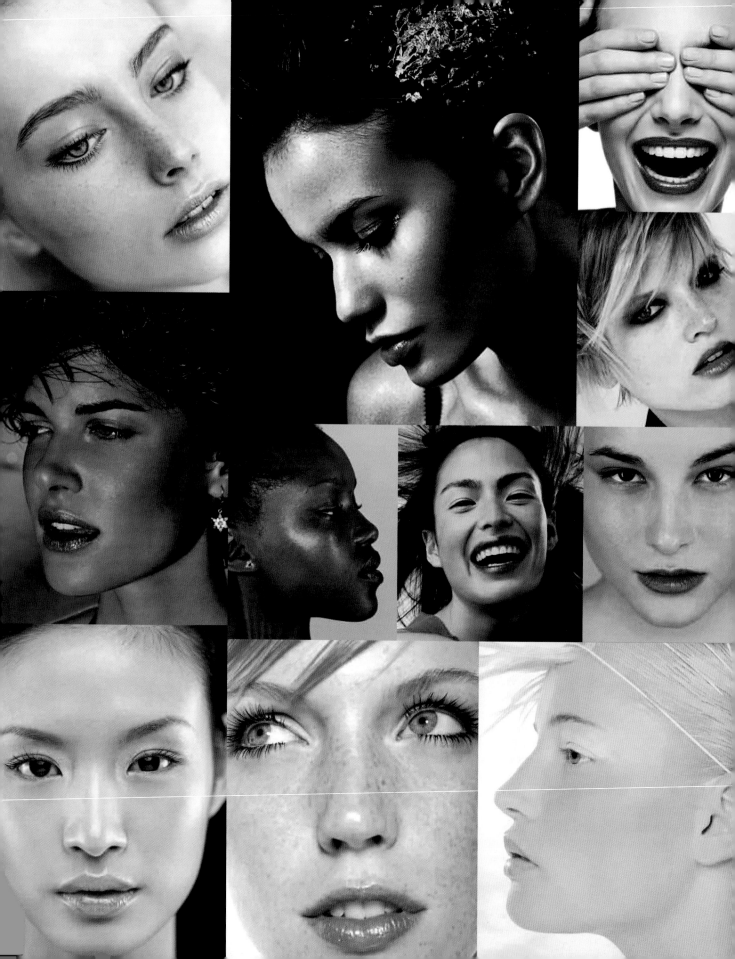

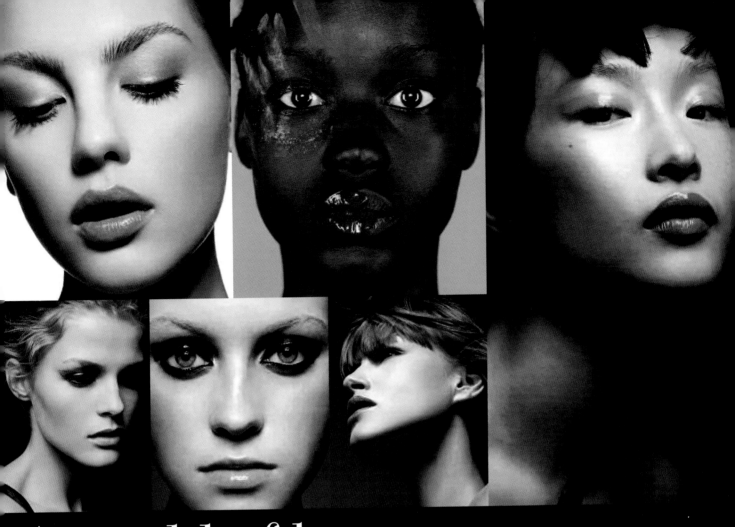

A world of beauty …

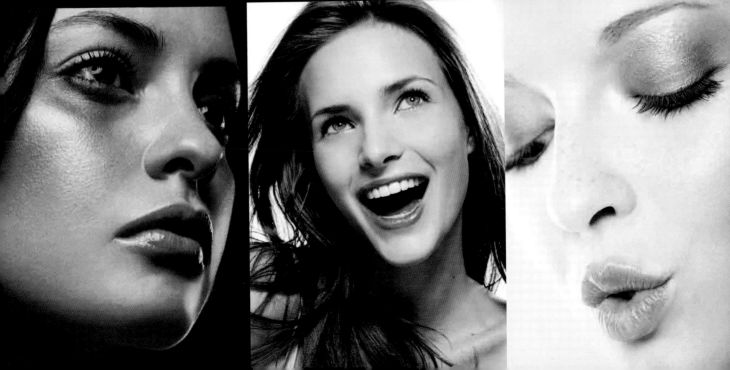

1 and you!

TAKING STOCK OF THE SKIN YOU'RE IN

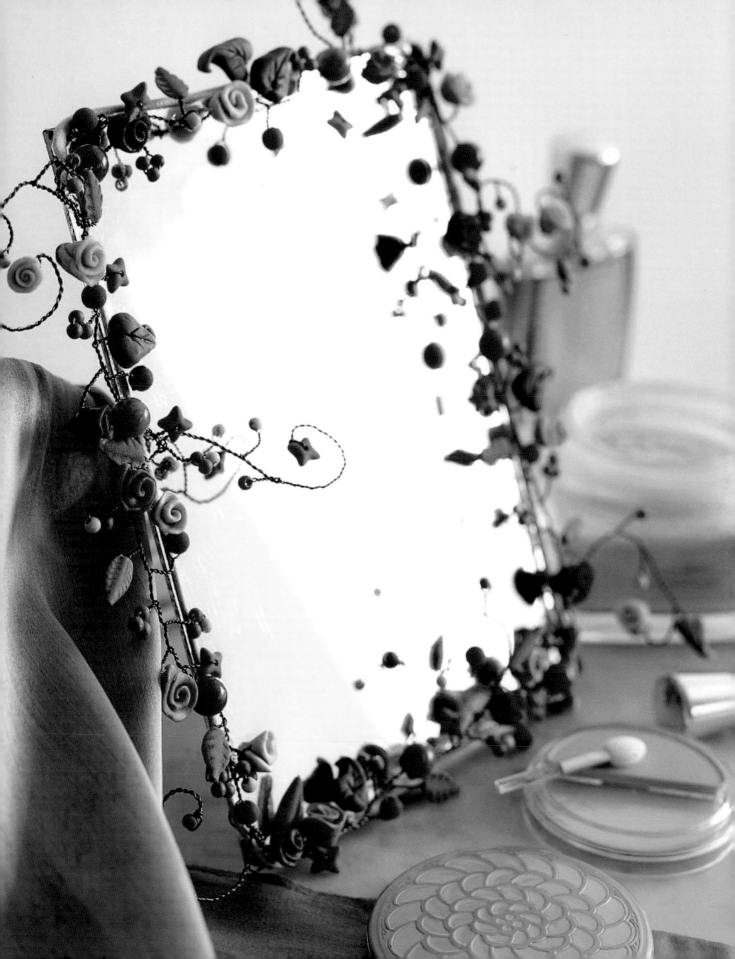

Fine-tuning any skin tone

From the fairest porcelain to the deepest tan, you can find a makeup palette that suits your skin tone. Here are some tips to get you on track ...

It's genetic: melanin, a natural pigment, is the primary determinant of human skin color or "phototype". There are ten basic tones used to classify white skin but over eighty for black skin! All light is reflected against "white" skin, making it lighter. On the other hand, the more melanin present, the more light the skin absorbs, producing an increasingly dark color.

FAIR Seasons and trends define your complexion: paleness — synonymous with freshness and purity — is back in style. You can accentuate milky skin without a heavy, masklike result. Out with monotony: pearly whites, translucent beige and rosy pinks afford deliciously sexy looks. Find the one that's right for you, whether your skin is on the pinkish side (look for rosy foundation and copper bronzing powder) or more yellowy (foundation in matching tones and gold-tone bronzing powder).

MEDIUM–GOLDEN Even if there's no mistaking that over-tanned skin is out, a sun-kissed complexion — completely natural or not — is the most effective face-lift out there. And today it's at your fingertips with an artful brushstroke. However, there is a world of nuances to discover between gold and copper ...

AMBER Mixed-race women must not let their wonderfully rich skin appear too yellowy. Opt for orange or rosy beige tones to emphasize fruity undertones.

BROWN TO BLACK Peach-toned correctors help brighten the darkest skin tones and capture light: small bursts of color enliven and give contour and vitality to your skin.

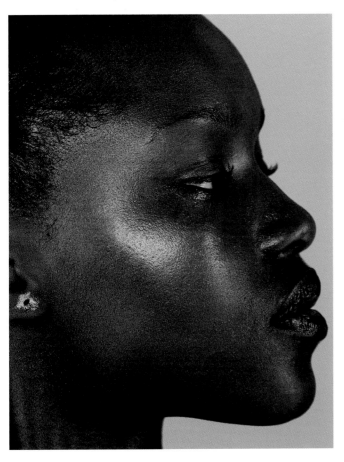
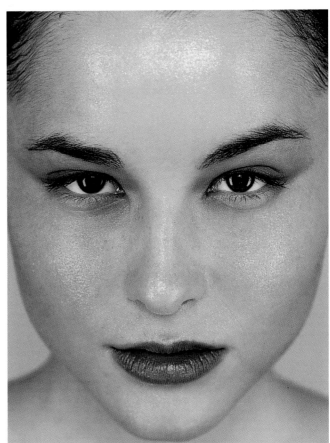
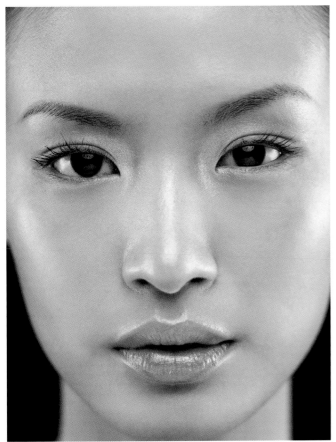
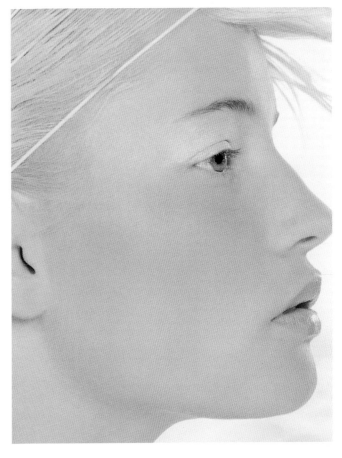

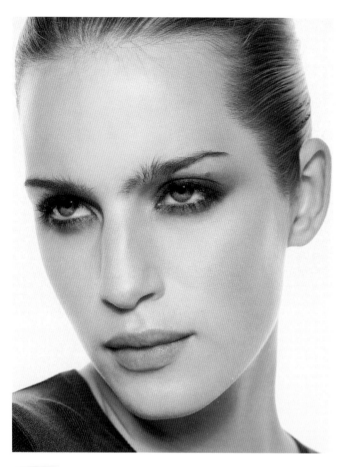
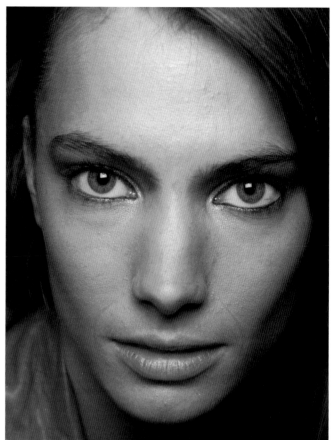
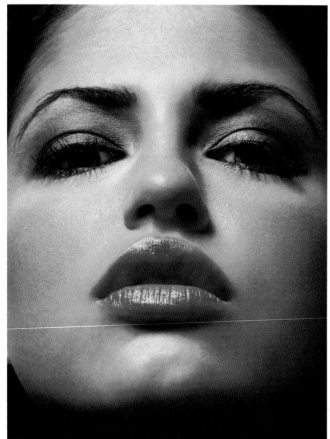
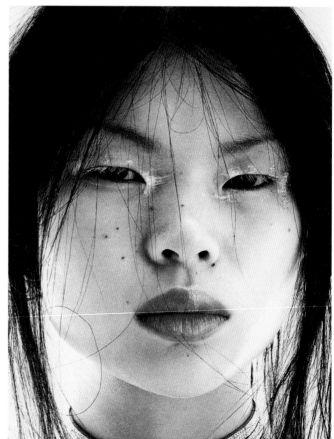

Know your facial structure

There is no place in today's world for antiquity's canonically perfect oval: an ideal facial architecture divided into three equal parts — forehead, nose and mouth. Long live diversity! One simple rule: be yourself and make the best of what you have.

OVAL Eyes separated by an eye's-length, a forehead wider than the lower face and eyebrows that arch just above the middle of your eyes: in a word, this is perfection. Use makeup to help bring out your personality by highlighting either your eyes or your lips.

RECTANGULAR Horizontal lines will help give your face more width and vivacity. Shorter and less-arched eyebrows will also help you attain this. Blush should always go below your cheekbones.

TRIANGULAR You can enhance the inherent femininity of a wide forehead and a small, narrower chin by accenting your cheekbones under well filled-out eyebrows.

SQUARE Sweeping your brush upward toward your temples can minimize a harsh jaw line and soften the lines of your face. Generous eyebrow shaping in the direction of the outer edge will also help.

ROUND It's all about creating an illusion of length... fuller cheeks tend to appear more slender with an upward application movement in your makeup. Use only very light colors and avoid all browns. Keep your eyebrows on the thick side and as tapered outwards as possible.

ANGULAR Makeup will help you smooth the edges. Drawing your eyebrows out toward your temples will somewhat soften geometric facial features.

ADVICE FROM A PROFESSIONAL MAKEUP ARTIST (Stila): Facial shapes can sometimes reveal character traits hidden even from oneself. Looking beyond structural categories, thankfully, no one is "average" and there can be no general rule for everybody. If you close your eyes and explore the unique curves and contours of your face, you will intuitively know what to accent, thanks to new formulas in today's cosmetics.

Your eye color

An erratic mirror of your emotions, a subtle palette that expresses the many nuances of your personality, a decisive weapon that you will be able to magnify through countless harmonies.

BLUE A marvelous optical illusion (the low quantities of melanin within the iris, coupled with the action of chromosome 15, reflect light much like a lake would) graces you with the most celebrated of eye colors. Take advantage of it, but without overdoing it. For titillating pupils, avoid combining blue-toned shadows in favor of warmer tones like navy, smoky gray, chocolate, apricot or copper.

GREEN Chromosome 19 affords you this pretty and rare eye color. From mauve to prune, all shades of red will add fire to your gaze: opposites attract, as they say.

GRAY A shade that can hide another and reflect your mood as well as the sky's. Want them to appear blue? Gray or coppery red will do the trick. Feeling green? Dress in lavender or aquamarine.

HAZEL Warm, sandy tones ranging from beige to brown and very dark eyelashes will complement these brilliant peepers, as will all prune, purple and green–bronze tones.

BLACK The rainbow's spectrum offers itself to you, but beware of too-light or pearly tones that can unflatteringly discolor the whites of your eyes. Midnight blue, dark gray, brown or buff tones will accentuate the mystery of dark eyes.

ADVICE FROM A PROFESSIONAL MAKEUP ARTIST (Stila):
How to choose between cooler (blue-toned) and warmer shades? All you need to do is hold a color up to your face in a mirror to determine if it boosts or busts. Depending on what you want to tone down, hide or unleash, play with harmony and discord between your eye color and your lips and cheeks.

It's genetic:
Once again, melanin levels define the color of your iris and, depending on how it's distributed, create a consistent shade, a dark ring on a light eye, or multi-colored flecks.

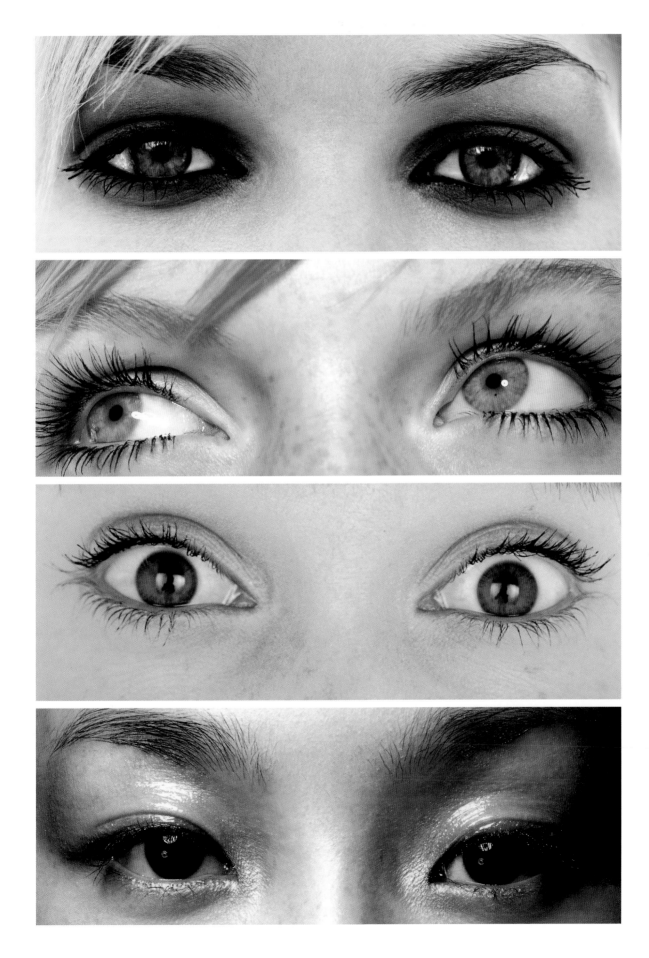

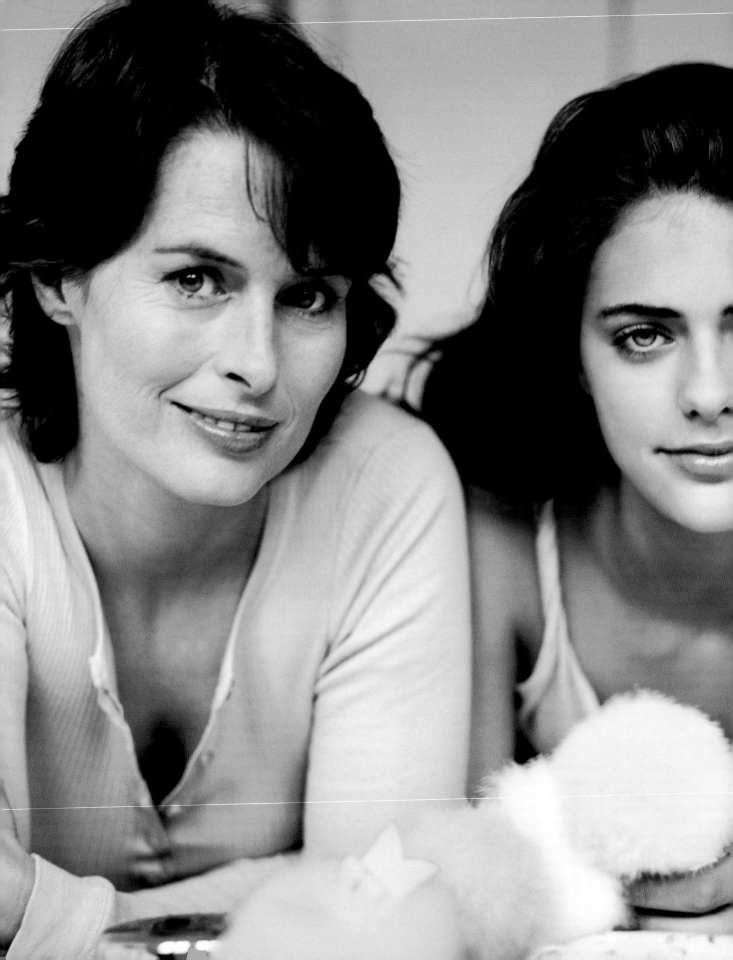

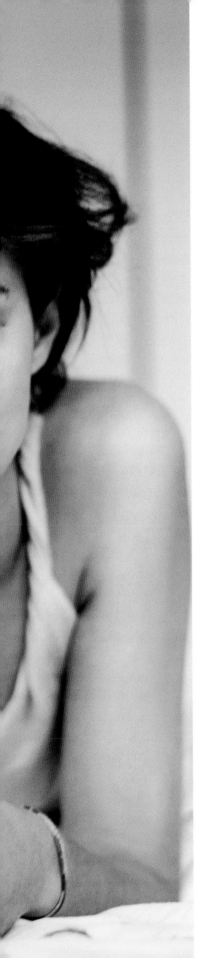

Gorgeous at twenty ... and at every age!

Growing old gracefully and effortlessly, rekindling your beauty at any age: today's cosmetic industry has integrated all this and more into products enhancing your natural look. A radiant example of mother–daughter mirror images.

The complicity between mother and daughter is at its height during a blissful beauty session at the spa. The generation gap is indeed closing, notably helped along by ever-increasing awareness of the importance of lifelong health and dietary consciousnesses, without forgetting the role played by cosmetics, the entire science of which is dedicated to lasting good looks.

THE NEW BREAKDOWN: YOUR BEAUTY REGIME

15–20 years old Know what you've got and take advantage of it.

30 years old You know what you want and what textures and formulas you prefer.

40 years old It's the dolce vita: refine a few things and rediscover yourself.

50 years old and beyond You want it all and like being surprised.

THE UNDER TWENTY DEPARTMENT

It's useless to swipe Mom's beauty products: this is the time to favor freshness and simplicity. At this age your assets are immense. Don't waste it by hiding under a layer of banality.

• Don't play with your eyebrows: losing their natural shape now could lead to long-term regrets.

COMPLEXION

• tinted moisturizer for a well-blended, even finish that won't clog your pores

• luminizing powder to cover up minor imperfections

• cheek stain that doubles as lip stain.

EYES

• pencils are undeniably the best tool at your age for gently treating your eyelids: less brutal than eyeliner, even (or rather especially) at the only age where your only wish is to grow older more quickly!

LIPS

• no need for artificial "plumping"; gloss or shine are by far preferable to an overdone lipstick. A beige or pink hydrating lip balm combines treatment and glam results.

FOCUS TEN YEARS ... LESS SPOTS TO BRIGHTEN UP

The secret: Use small bursts of effective highlighting like the fashion-industry professionals who make actresses look their best onscreen.

Direct light on your face can accentuate any dark circles under your eyes — we all know how cruel and revealing overhead lighting can be on our danger zones. On the other hand, makeup will help you brighten these strategic spots:

• nasolabial folds — the creases that run from your nose to the corners of your mouth

• "lion" wrinkles — between the eyebrows

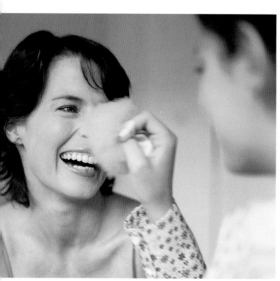

Powder puff pointers
Mastering powder application is an art: as long as you apply it with the lightness of a feather, the velvety or matte look it affords will greatly enhance your skin. Restricting its application to the middle of the face will guarantee a vivacious finish and not paralyze your expression — which should remain the absolute priority.

• inner corners of your eyes

• eyelid crease

• contours of your mouth.

AS YOU GET OLDER, GO EASY!

FOUNDATION

Foundation is to be used with caution: as the face grows older, it needs more light but certainly not more thickness. New formulas that let your skin breath and add radiance will give you a professional look without being too heavy. A mix of concealer and foundation, always a half-tone lighter than your skin, will sweep away shadows from:

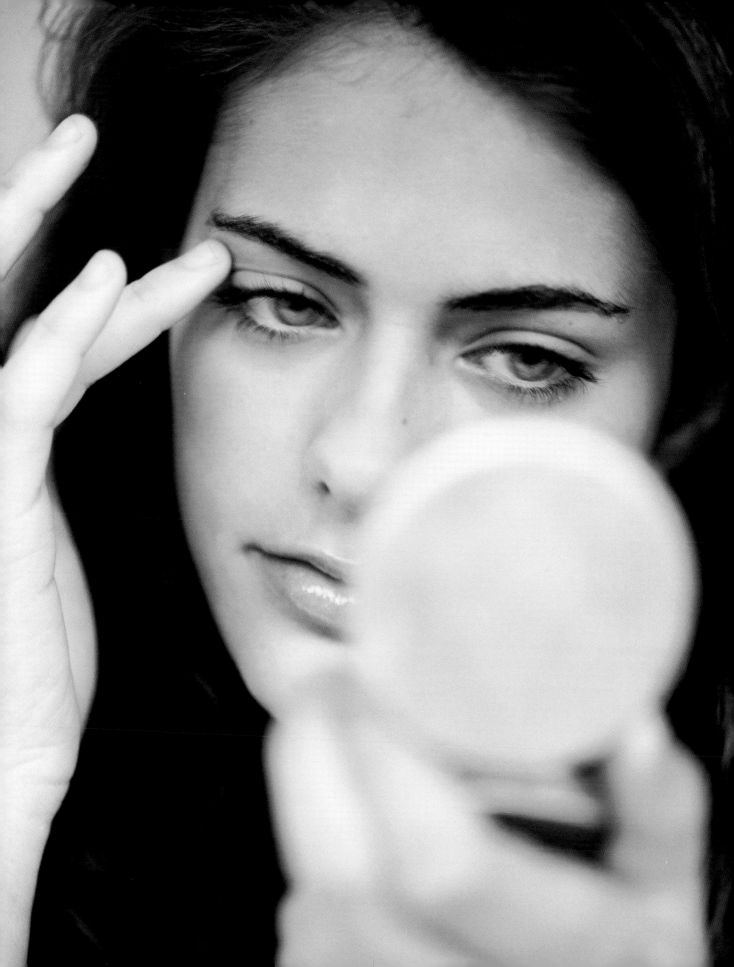

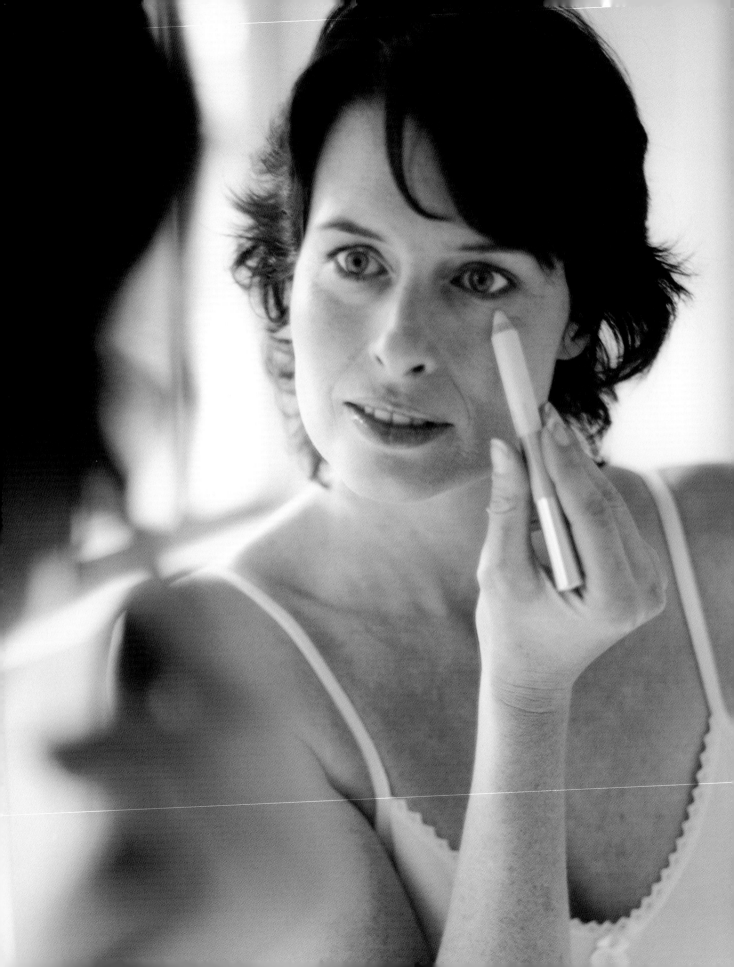

- the inner corners of your eyes
- the creases running from the nose to the corner of the mouth
- the contours of the mouth
- below the lower lip.

A concealer stick used sparingly will cover minor flaws but be careful to only spot where necessary and aim for natural coverage. Beware of overdoing it and plastering on a crescent under your eye!

- Nothing is better than ice cubes to liven up your complexion and stimulate your lymphatic system. But always put ice in a towel to avoid burning your skin.

LIPS

- Plumping effect guaranteed: use a moisturizing balm and a lip contour treatment. Leave it on as long as possible to hydrate lips and banish small wrinkles.
- Lip shaping pencil: opt for a fat tip and follow the outer edge. Don't use on the corners of your lips to avoid caking.
- Pearly pink eye shadow can be used as a gloss in combination with a red semi-gloss.

EYES

- Beware of overdoing your eye shadow: powder can build up in the small expressive wrinkles around the eyes, making them much more visible than without any makeup!
- Blue eyedrops make your eyes brighter and fresher looking
- Dusky, matte shadows bring out the sparkle in your eyes
- Accentuate your eyebrow form — thinning and lightening are the first sign of age. Fill them in towards your temples.
- A thin line of off-white kohl pencil will make your eyes look bigger and prevent yellowish reflections on the cornea.
- Brown or gray mascara is less aggressive and just as dramatic as black.

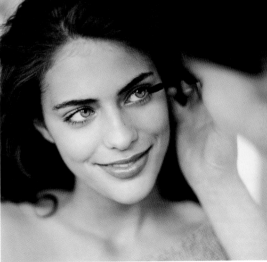

A single coat of mascara: and you're good to go!

Staying beautiful ...
today and tomorrow

A clear lipstick that takes on the color of your dreams? A "perfect skin" pill? Special-effect products that add light from within? Long live science! Here's a rundown of what's in store in the future with biologist Gérard Redziniak (Pacific Creation).

Tomorrow's mirror just might be a computer with a built-in camera that will manage your colors according to your mood or a particular celebrity look that you want to create on a given day. **Laser technology** will help you pick the best mascara or identify and banish problem wrinkles before they develop. Biology and cosmetic science will unite to create clarifiers and concealers that will afford you flawless skin. **Absolute moisturizers** and **second-skin formulas** will be commonplace, as will infinitely natural-looking masks. Light-diffusing, soft focus complexion enhancers will make light bounce off the skin according to the angle it shines on you. **Clear liquid crystals like those in LCD screens will** enhance this "radiance" and reflect **dazzlingly magnificent colors** using Polaroid techniques where invisible particles protect your skin while giving off a suntanned look. We'll be chameleons with makeup that is self-adapting to our surroundings and the circumstances. "Smart" foundations will identify problem areas and correct them before they become visible. An **utterly clear lipstick** whose active ingredients will morph **from the sheerest gloss to the deepest red** with an infinite range of possibilities in respect to available light will instantly generate a **protective polymer plumping film** directly on the lips. You decide between simple and natural or the most theatrical looks imaginable. Chemistry will also help by creating freeze drying techniques yielding extremely pure powders. Or with molecular encapsulation producing sun screens and dyes locked in miniscule glass pearls that never come into direct contact with the skin: a limitless color palette at your fingertips, prohibited today because of toxicity. Polymers and other **microscopic particles, such as mini light tubes or diodes that illuminate your skin for an evening,** will highlight specific features. Finally, we'll give off an aura of diamonds without even needing to pierce our ears ...

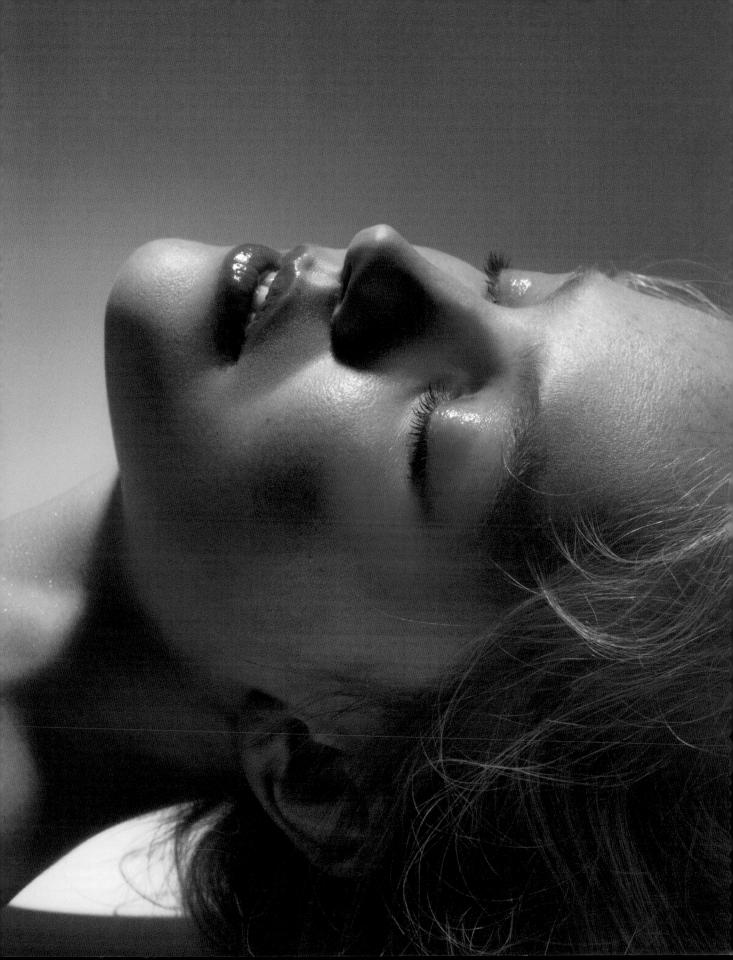

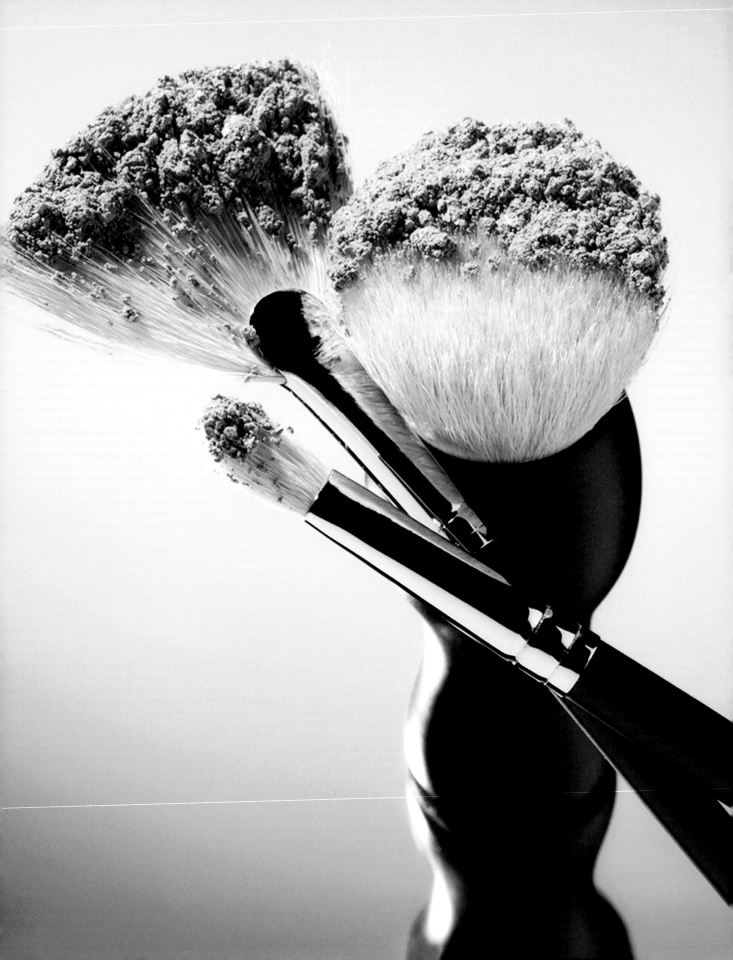

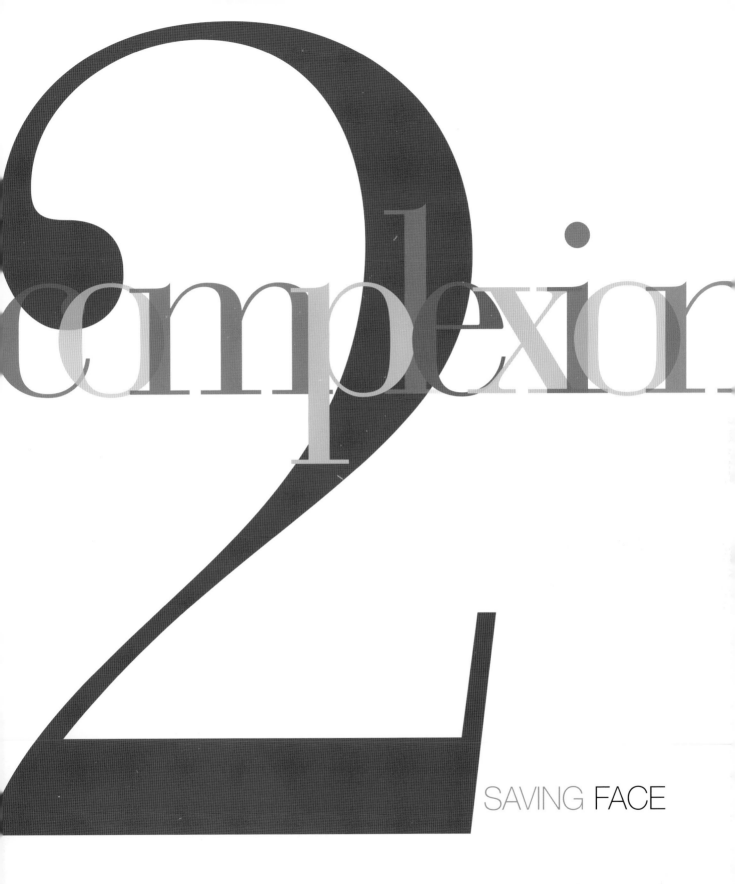

2

complexion

SAVING FACE

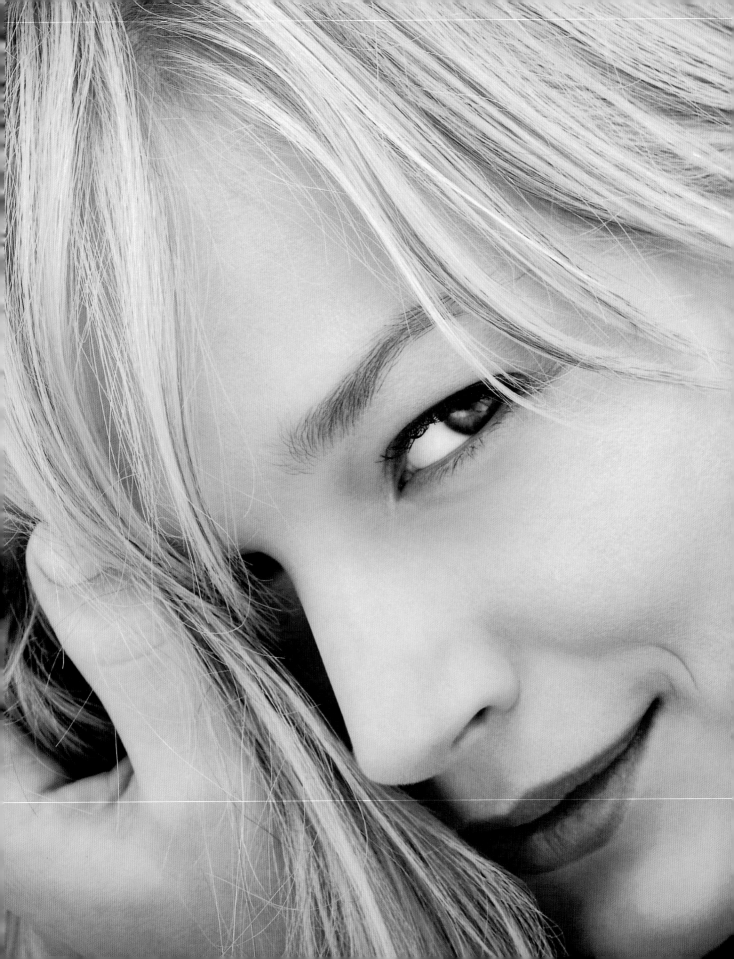

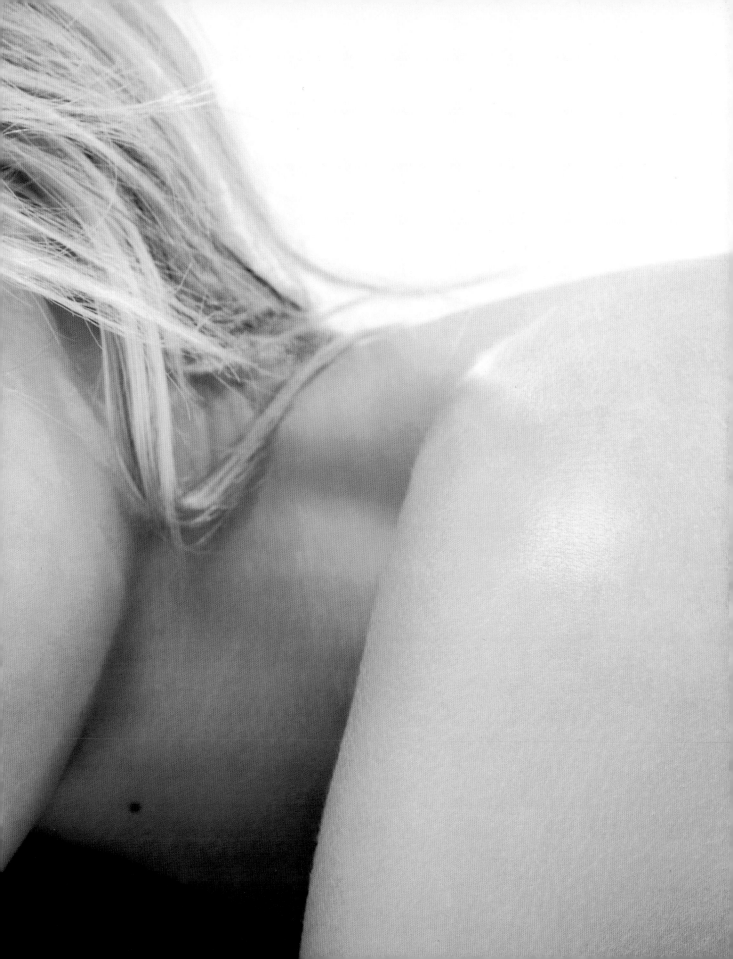

•Infinitely beige: naturally sheer, sublimely discreet.

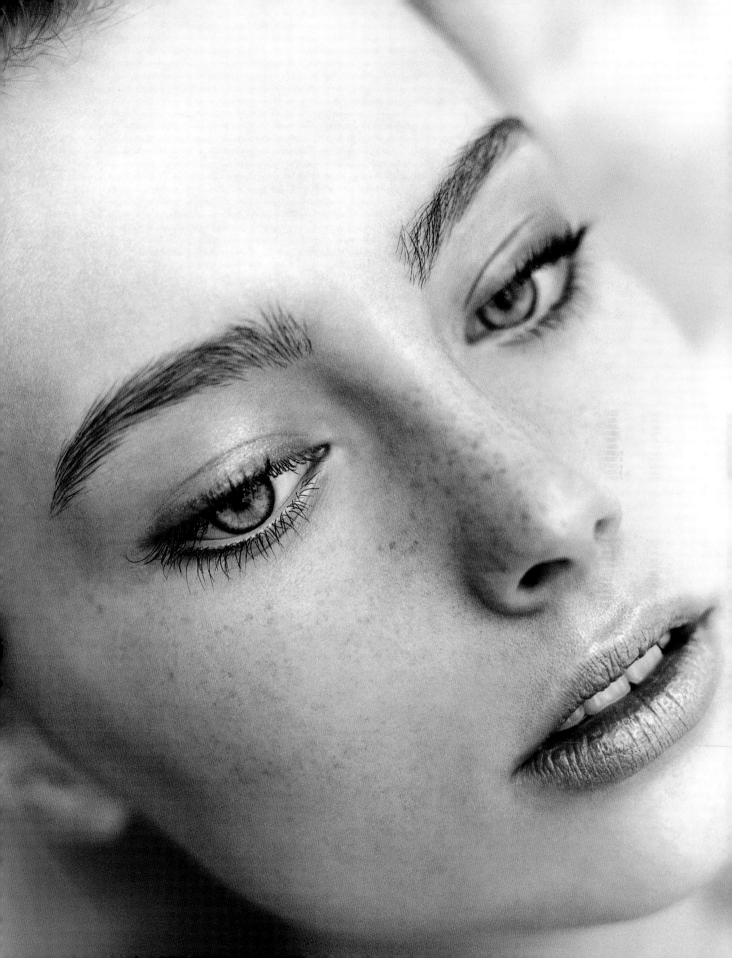

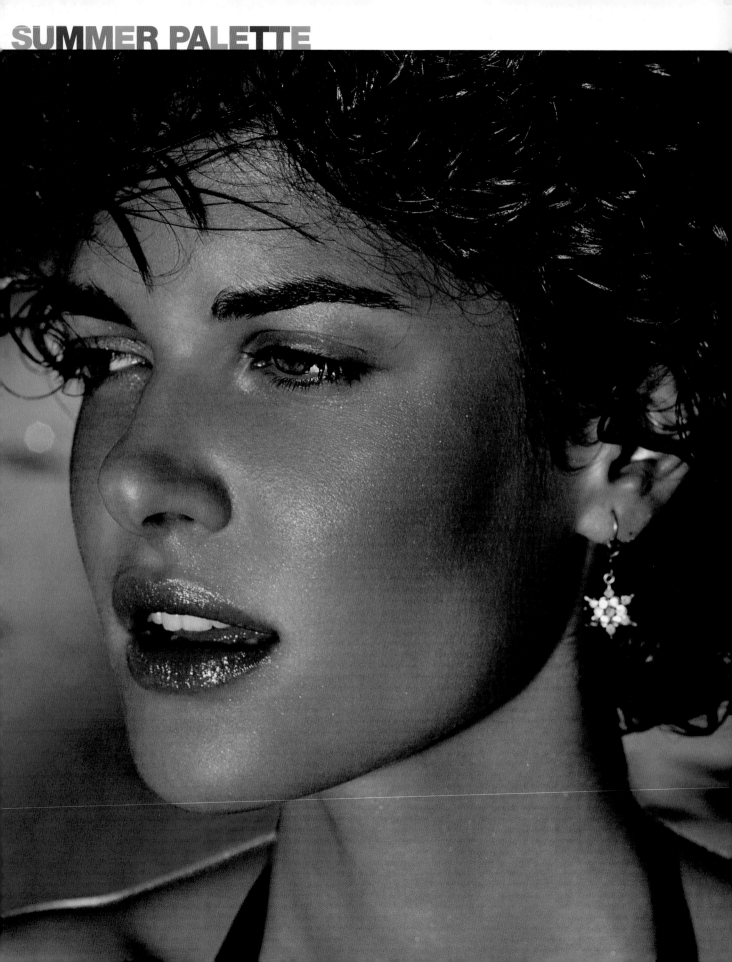

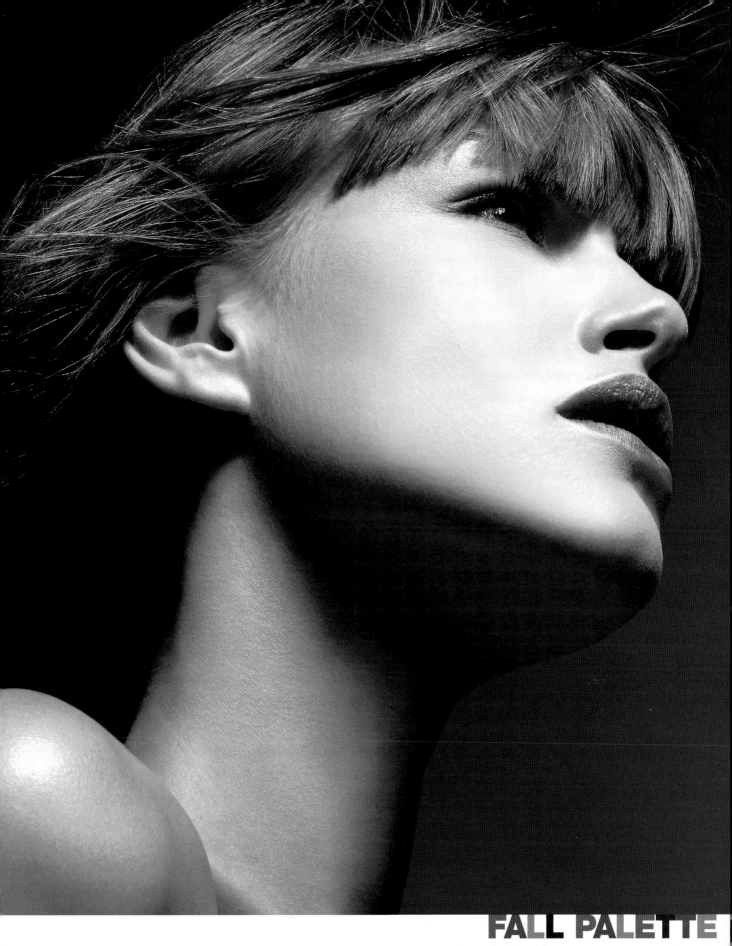

FALL PALETTE

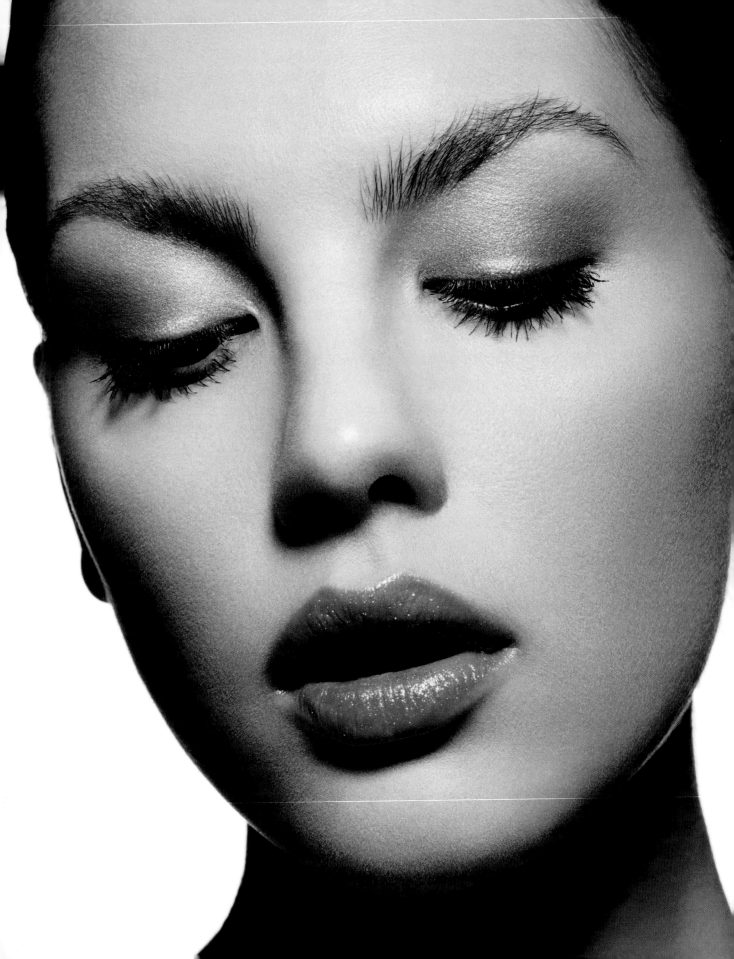

Like snow flakes and rose petals...

Bare skin: the real you

Of the four basic skin types, knowing which is yours is essential in choosing the products that are right for you. The basics for feeling good ... in the skin you're in!

FAIR SKIN

...normal to dry An ideally balanced Ph level explains the finesse of your skin's soft, supple grain. This is a precious asset that you must protect from the ravages of time or the environment. Once correctly cleansed, scrubbed, moisturized and protected (notably from the sun's harming rays), your face will be the perfect canvas to showcase your beauty, day in, day out.

...dry to very dry Enemies of your translucent yet ultra-sensitive and fragile skin abound. Temperature extremes, pollution ... and ageing all contribute to premature wrinkles and rosacea blotches. Your top priorities: nourish and moisturize. Eighty percent of women with this skin type don't do enough in this department. Why not try out the benefits of a humidifier?

...oily skin is generally thicker and more resistant to pollutants, damage ... and even age! Main concerns are combating shine, evening out dilated pores and fighting blackheads and breakouts. Dilated pores can also complicate makeup application. Keep a close eye on your diet and hygiene and consider hormone therapy.

DARK SKIN Positive factors include a high concentration of collagen and elastin (that helps curb the ageing process) coupled with an acidic Ph and fifteen layers of sun-blocking keratin from head to toe. Makeup application and maintenance is complicated, however, by perspiration and high sebum production. Your skin requires the same treatments as blotchy fair complexions.

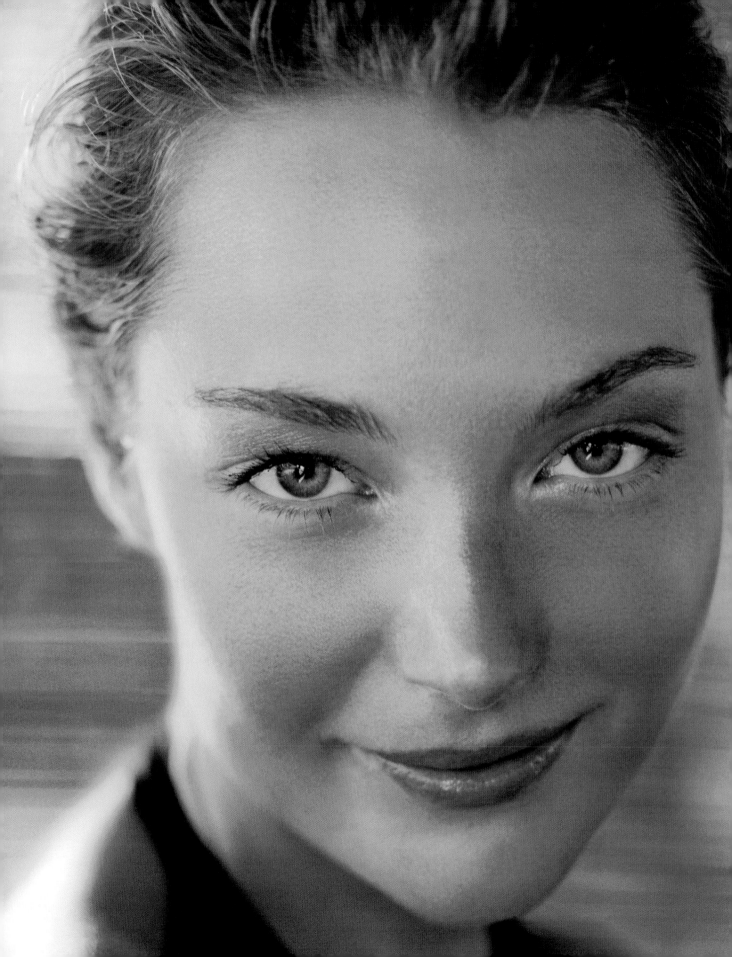

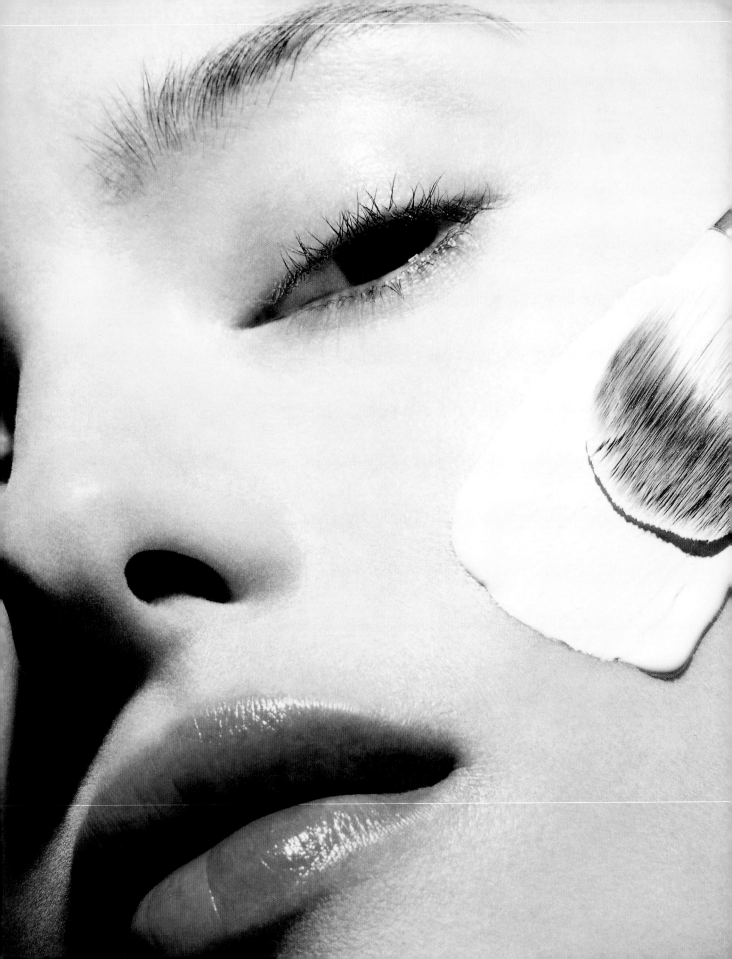

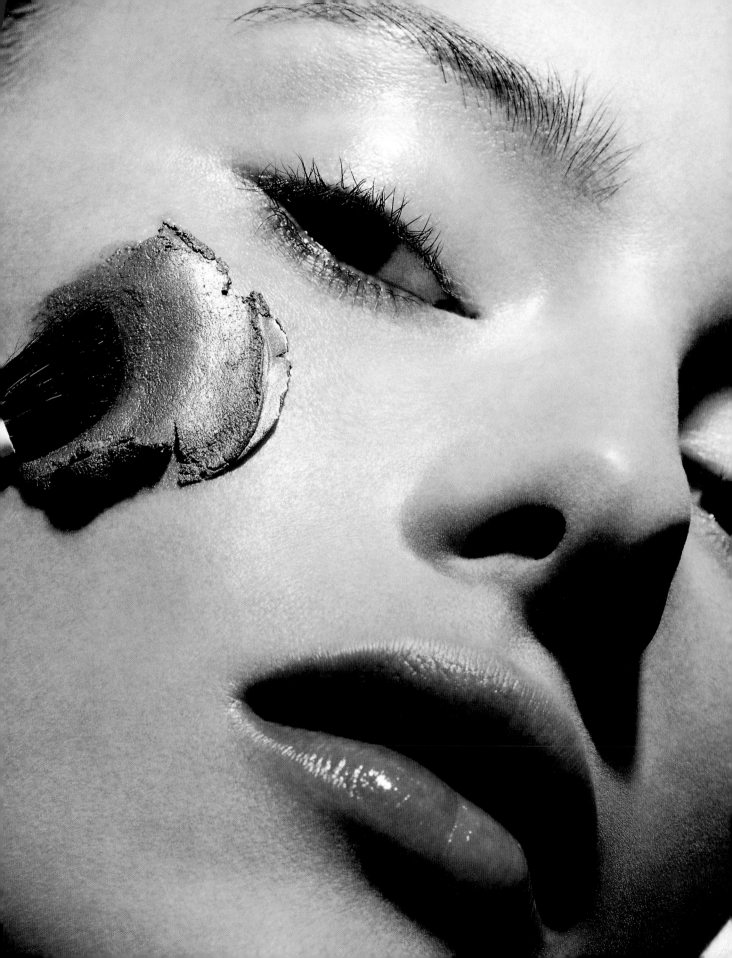

Mission: beautiful skin, zero flaws

*You can achieve any look you want …
as long as your bases are covered.
A canvas of impeccable skin is key.*

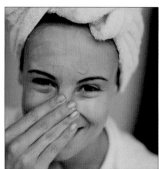

EVERY MORNING: MOISTURIZE AND PURIFY

• Proper moisturizing starts with a large glass of water straight of out bed • wipe your face with a well-drenched towelette in the morning (lotion adapted to your skin type or mineral water) • use a cotton swab to clean the inner corners of your eyes and remove any traces of mascara or makeup remover on your lashes • use a tissue to absorb any extra moisture — paradoxically, skin that stays wet dries out more quickly • check that your eyebrows are well-tweezed and relentlessly go after any strays.

MASSAGE AND EVEN OUT

The first step to bright skin is proper preparation • put a nickel-sized amount of lotion in the palm of your hand and perform a delicate yet vigorous massage in order to soften lines and increase the effectiveness of your moisturizers. "Warming up" your skin through circular and upward movements will help your day cream penetrate deeper and guarantee ideal moisturizing, prepping your skin for minimal makeup and maximum effect. Once microcirculation is stimulated, your skin breathes better … and it shows! • don't limit your moisturizer to your face: lavish your neck and shoulders with hydrating creams, being sure to always blend upwards.

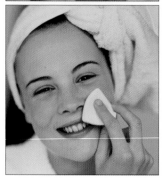

ADVICE FROM A PROFESSIONAL MAKEUP ARTIST (Stila)
Your face is a canvas that needs to be wiped clean every day. Exfoliating helps remove all the small yet toxic intruders of everyday life, such as climate or stress-related imperfections, dry spots, small pimples or other blotches, and is a quick way to calm and restore your complexion.

Exfoliate once a week
Using a mild exfoliant once a week is the only way to remove dead skin cells and to avoid looking ashen. Follow up with a facial.

5-minute Express Beauty
Envelop your face in a towel filled with ice cubes.

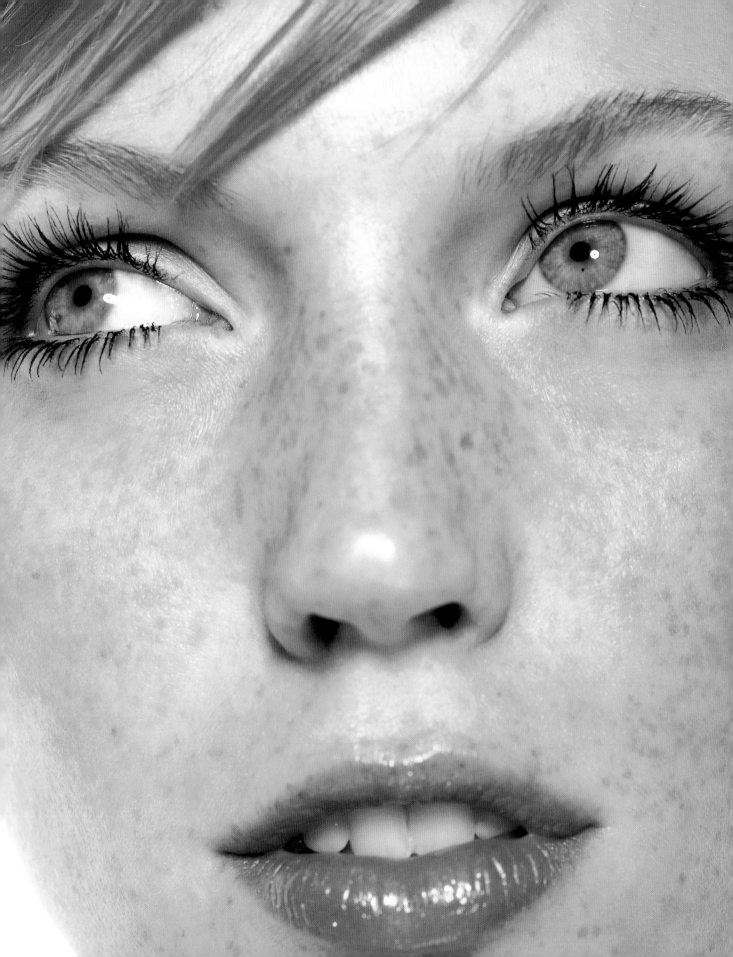

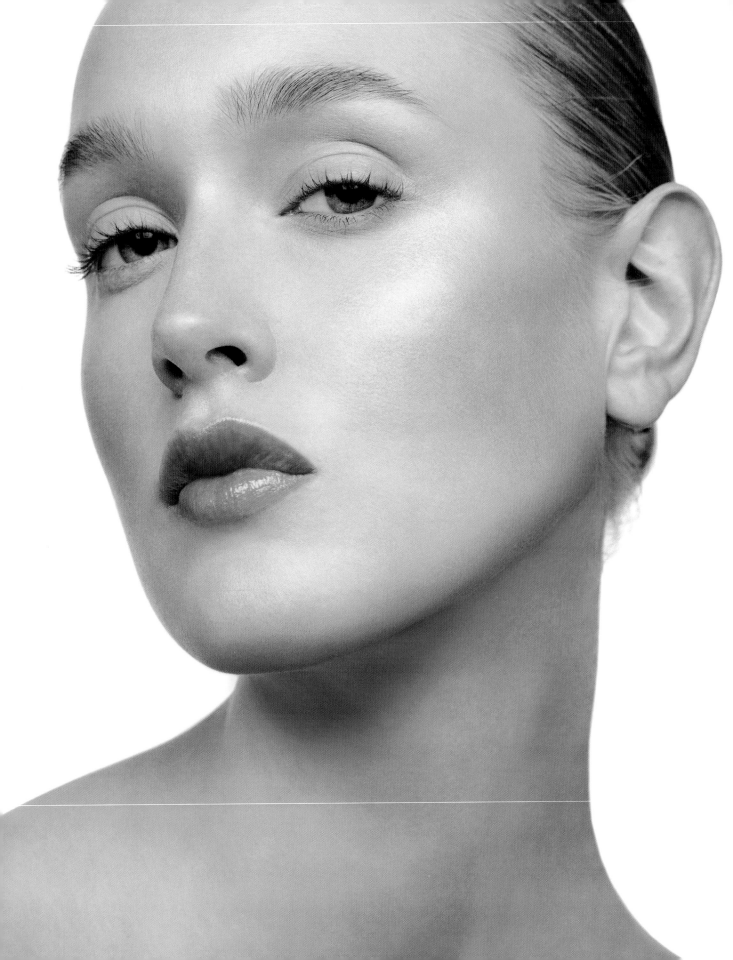

Touching base: capturing the light

A glowing complexion that brilliantly reflects all the facets of your personality: complexion enhancers have reinvented skin science and have become standards in beauty.

COMPLEXION ILLUMINIZERS, ENHANCERS, VEIL OF LIGHT It's to skin what gloss is to lips, a new generation of products that brilliantly keep their promise: they contain pearly pigments that reflect and diffuse ambient light to give your skin a radiant glow and make it anything but lackluster.

USE alone, or for more spectacular effects, coupled with a classic foundation — the two can be easily blended if their respective consistency allows. The result is a perfectly luminous base.

CHOOSE beige tones for pale complexions or muted apricot tones for more golden skin. Place a dot on the back of your hand and pass the brush through it before applying a very small amount to the middle of your eyelid, the bridge of your nose and the top of your cheekbones. It will capture the light and your skin will be radiant as a result.

FOR MAXIMUM LUSTER you can also use it, after foundation for a final touch, on your cheekbones, nose, chin, brow bone and your hairline.

To replump your lips and hold lipstick in place: blend up to the lip line before applying lip color.

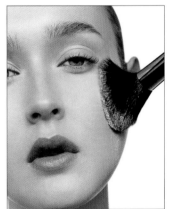

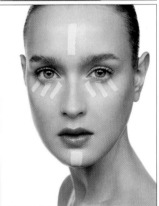

The magic line: center of the forehead, bridge of the nose, tip of the chin and top of the cheekbones

What you'll need
- a full brush
- nimble fingers!

Concealer: a no-stress antidote to dull skin

An all-purpose product that hides, disguises, corrects, and gives a flawless matt finish. Impossible to live without, you should find the one that's right for you.

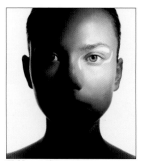

Effect 1
Light up your face

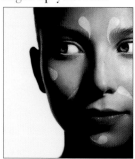

Effect 2
Highlight your features

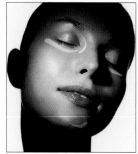

Effect 3
Hide imperfections

THE RIGHT COLOR: Concealer must be perfectly identical to your skin tone. The name of the game is flawless blending with your natural skin color to achieve absolute homogeny. It may be advisable to try two shades lighter than your skin since concealer changes colors rapidly. Optical pigments and light diffusers: makeup light years away from the plastering effects of its predecessors!

IN THE BAG OR NOT Whether or not you have dark circles, concealer simultaneously smoothes the skin under your eye, diminishes wrinkles, erases blood vessels along your nose and brightens your eyes at their inner corner or on the top of your eyelid.

Concealer also covers unfortunate pimples and softens the lines between your eyebrows. It adds radiance to your smile at the corners of your mouth, rubs out the "bitter wrinkles" and reduces shine on the tip of your nose.

APPLY always with vertical sweeps aided by small patting gestures, using a small brush — an easily procurable tool of the pros — for blending.

ADVICE FROM OLIVIER ECHAUDEMAISON (Guerlain)
Looking tired? A spot of concealer on each earlobe: who would have known, a surefire way to rejuvenate your look!

How to cover a pimple:
Use concealer a half shade lighter than your skin. Apply directly on the pimple, and don't forget to use powder to keep the product in place.

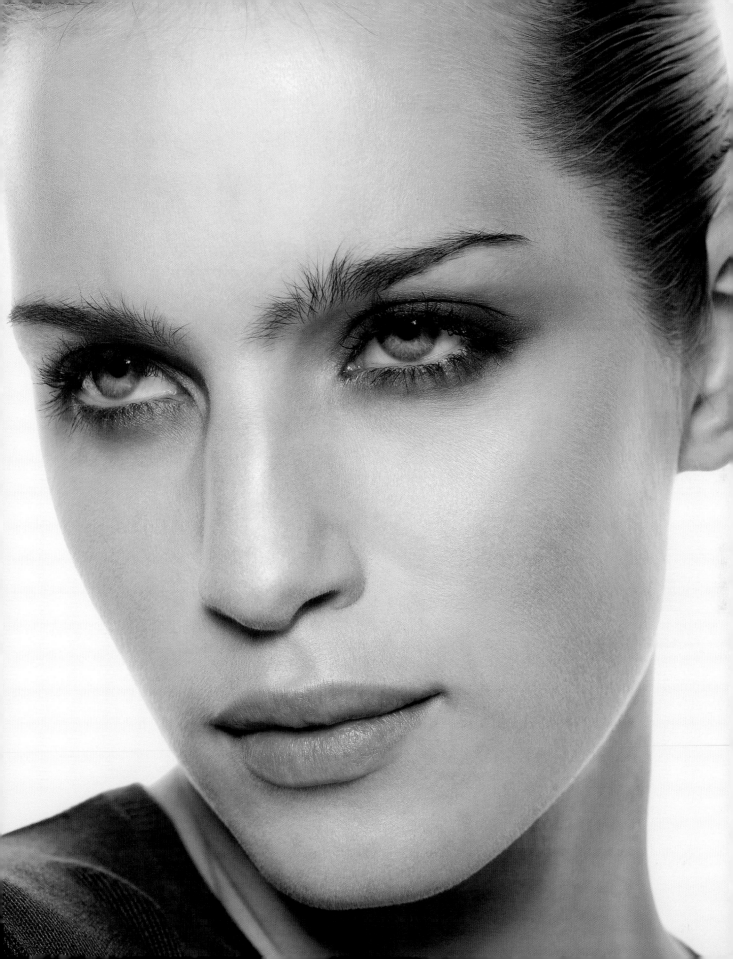

Foundation: at its lightest

Mastering the art of blending formulas and textures to silky smoothness, just the right shade and complete discretion: in a word, foundation is not what it used to be!

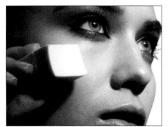

Freshness tip:
Use a latex makeup sponge imbibed with lotion to blend your foundation.

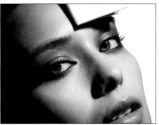

Beware of the T-Zone!
To avoid shine, gently pat your forehead, nose bridge and chin with a tissue.

Available in **stick** (better coverage and more practical application) or **liquid** form, a foundation that is in opposition to your skin type will paradoxically have the most in common with it! For dry skin you need a rich and satiny foundation. If your skin is oily, you'll need something lighter and smoother with a matte finish. Today's foundations let skin breathe, moisturize, protect from pollution and some even have anti-ageing properties. What more could you ask for?

SHADES Test along your jawline and opt for one tone lighter than your skin. You want to aim for unifying your complexion, not changing it. You don't want to run the risk of unsightly streaks.

If you use your **FINGERTIPS** to apply foundation, use a massaging motion to tonify and for perfect, smooth blending into your skin.

With a dry **FLAT BRUSH** (the fuller the brush, the easier the application) or a slightly damp **MAKEUP SPONGE**, you must be nimble as you pat it on, pay close attention to the contours of your eyes where buildup can lead to the one bad effect of poorly applied foundation: accentuated wrinkles. Apply, starting in the center of your face and blend outwards for the best effect.

ADVICE FROM A PROFESSIONAL MAKEUP ARTIST (Stila):
Choose according to the textre of your skin or your lifestyle — we like certain formulas just as we like certain drinks; we know what feels good against our skin. To get a "feeling" for a particular product, place a small amount on the top of your hand and warm it up with your fingertips before applying it to your face.

Tip for longer hold
Spraying lotion through a tissue will fix your foundation.

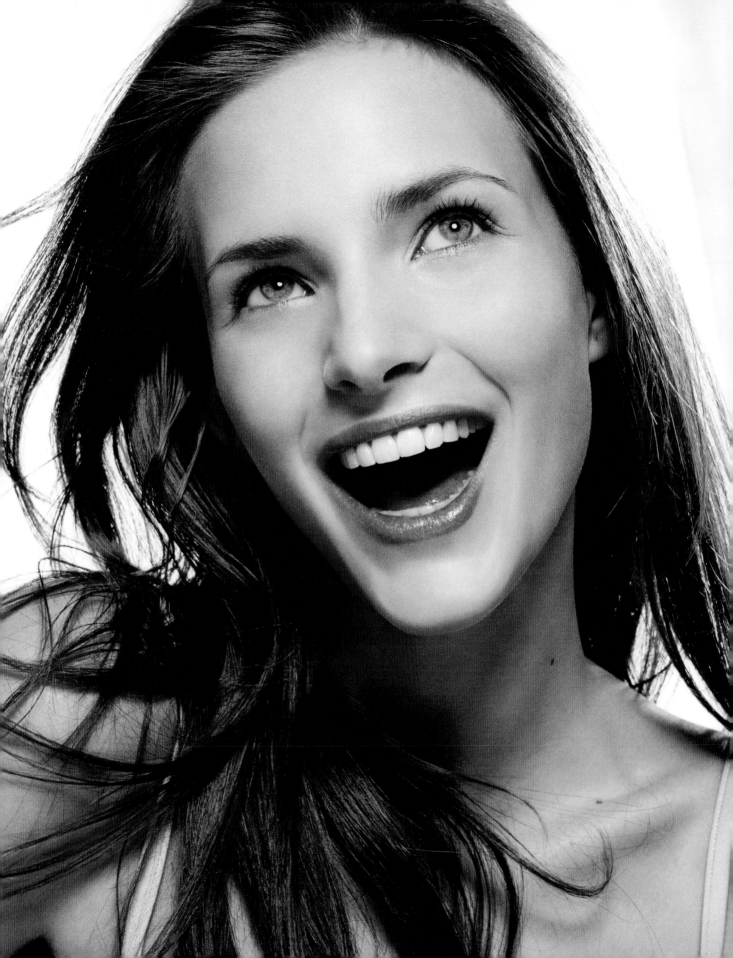

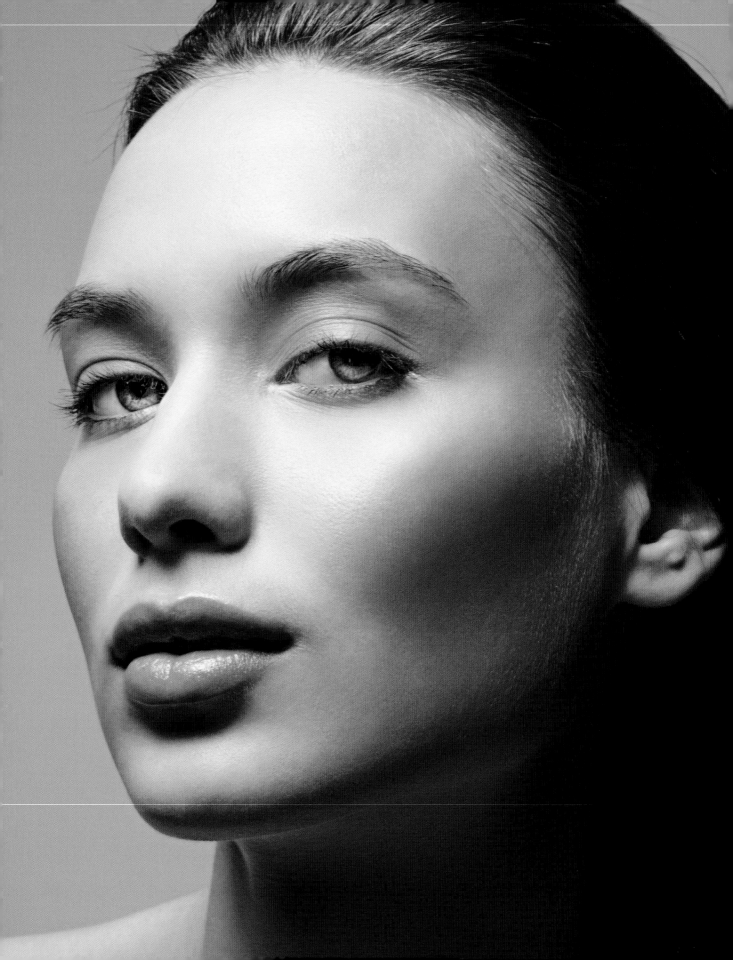

Bluffing with blush

For cheeks as fresh as after an early-morning walk or as expressive as a rush of emotion: blush is the final touch for getting your face in place

LOCATION IS EVERYTHING The shape of your face is your guide. You can sculpt round cheeks (start at the top of your ear, work your way down in a crescent motion until below your cheekbones), soften a square-like appearance (apply close to the ear and blend towards the cheekbones) or counter a rectangular facial structure (apply horizontally on cheekbones).

COLOR CODES Fair-skinned women should use lively pinks and reds. Darker-skinned women should opt for browns and corals. Tender roses, on the other hand, suit everyone!

Your **BRUSH** should not be too full to ensure blending of these micronized and condensed powders. You're looking for a range of colors that's worlds apart from the "trowel" effect.

Your **FINGERTIPS** can be used with inventive mousse or cream formulas that become powdery after application and present none of the hassle of their traditional, oilier counterparts. Dab the product on with your index finger for the right dose, and blend from your jaw to the cheekbone.

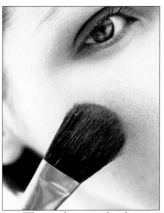

The right powder brings light to your eyelids and adds radiance to your face.

What you'll need:
- blush brush
- cream blush
- powder blush

The sun factor: carefree tanning tips

Self-tanners are both the most flattering and the most dangerous of inventions: it's a technique that requires the nimblest of fingers!

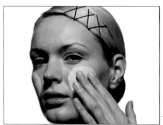
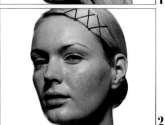
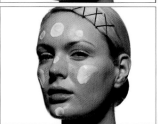
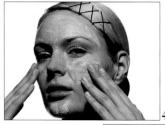
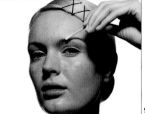

1 FOR A PERFECTLY UNIFORM TAN always start fresh: make sure you've used a gentle exfoliant (biological or mechanical) to remove all dead skin cells.

2 WELL MOISTURIZED SKIN is even more important when self-tanning since DHA (the principal component of self-tanners) has a tendency to dry skin out by draining water from skin cells.

3 TREAD WITH A LIGHT TOUCH: apply small amounts to your forehead, cheeks and chin — all the places the sun would affect first — without forgetting your ears and neck, blending towards your shoulders.

4 SPREAD self-tanners uniformly but quickly across your face by massaging with the flats of your fingers. And don't wait to wash your hands (and nails) vigorously with soap and water.

5 TO AVOID AN ORANGEY LOOK, which is always preferable, immediately after application wipe a cotton swab or a damp paper towel across your eyebrows and along your hairline.

ADVICE FROM ALINE SCHMITT (studio makeup artist): Wait 15 minutes before applying makeup after using a self-tanner. Your foundation will tone down while your self-tanner will kick in!

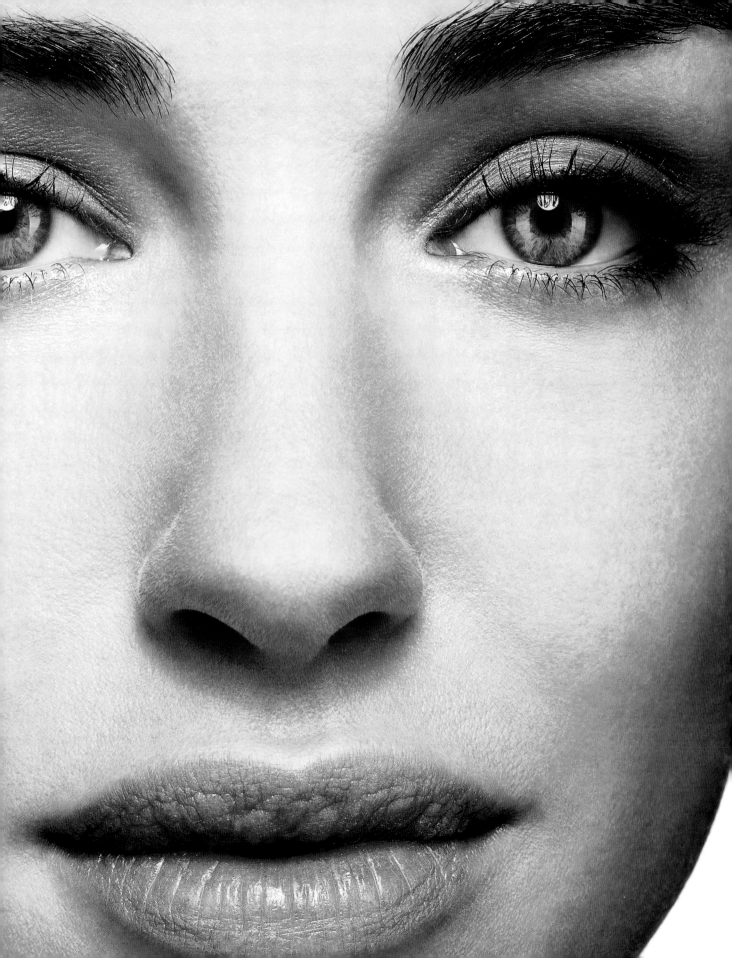

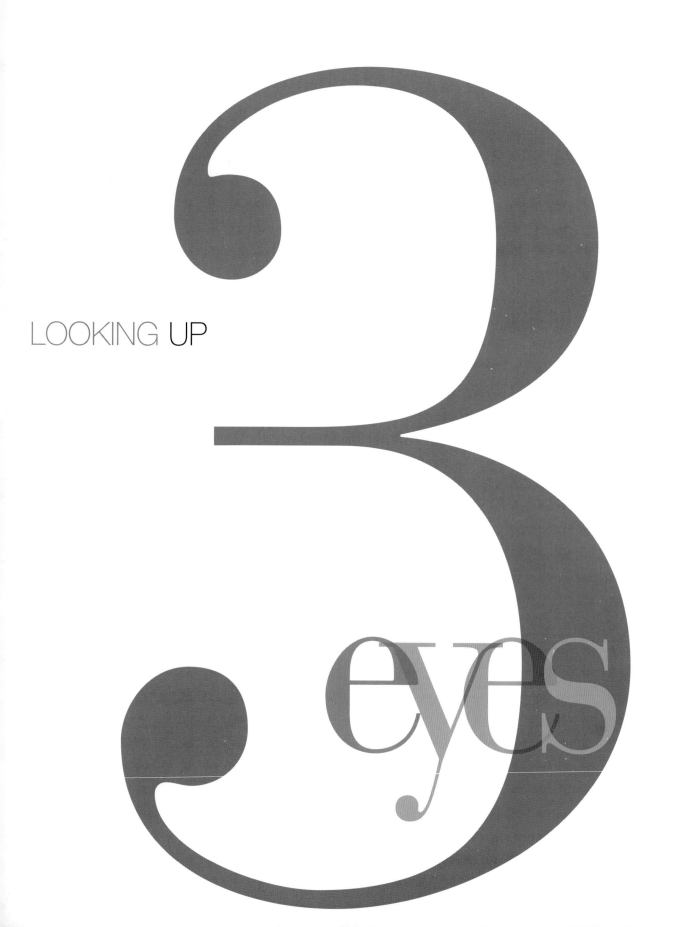

LOOKING UP

3

eyes

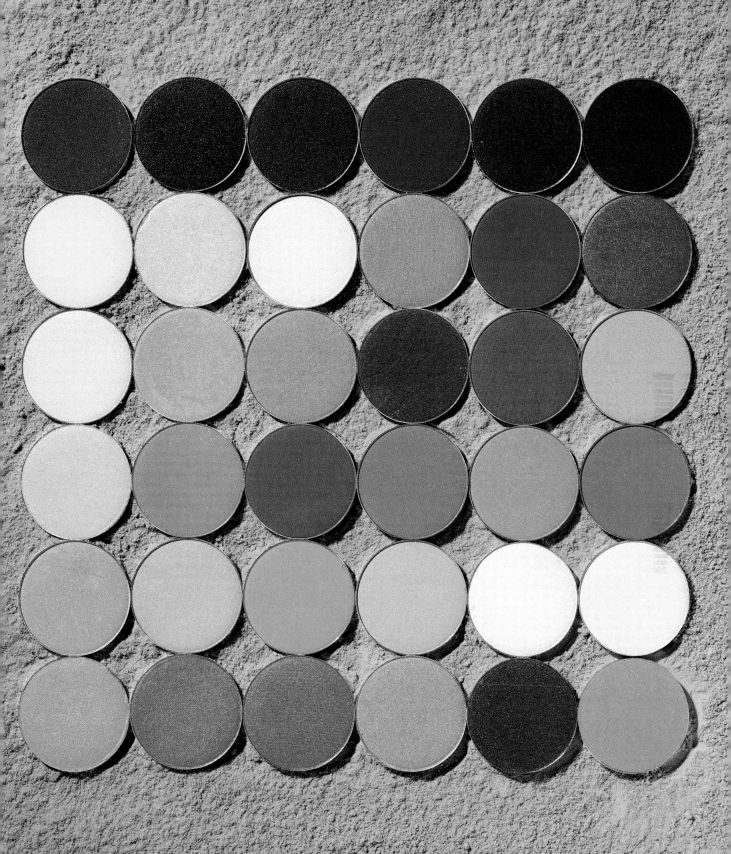

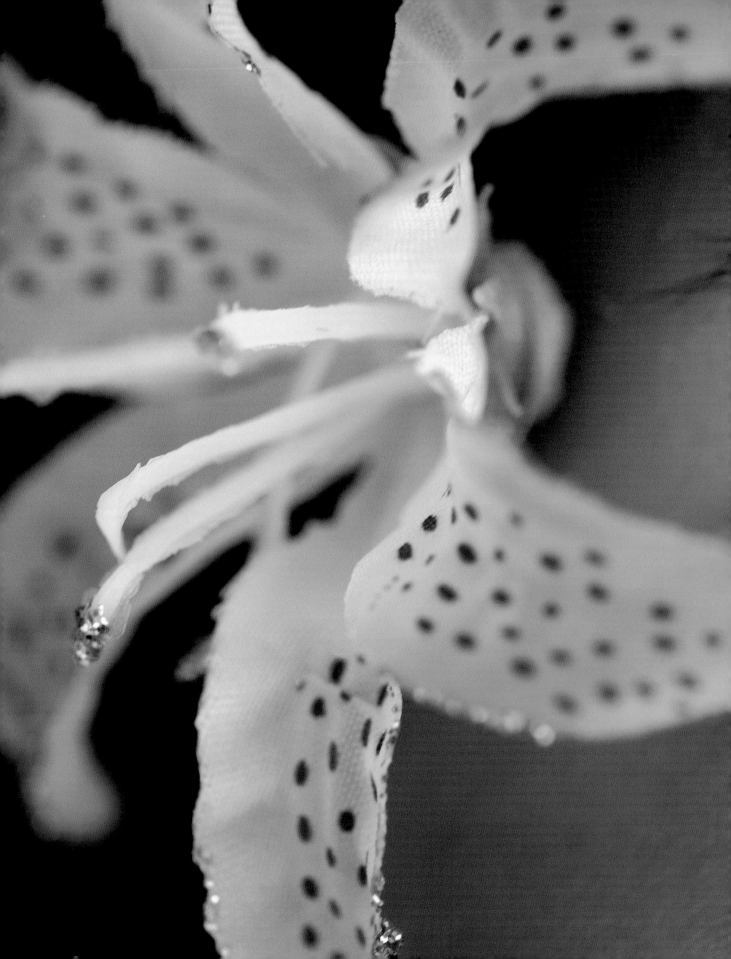

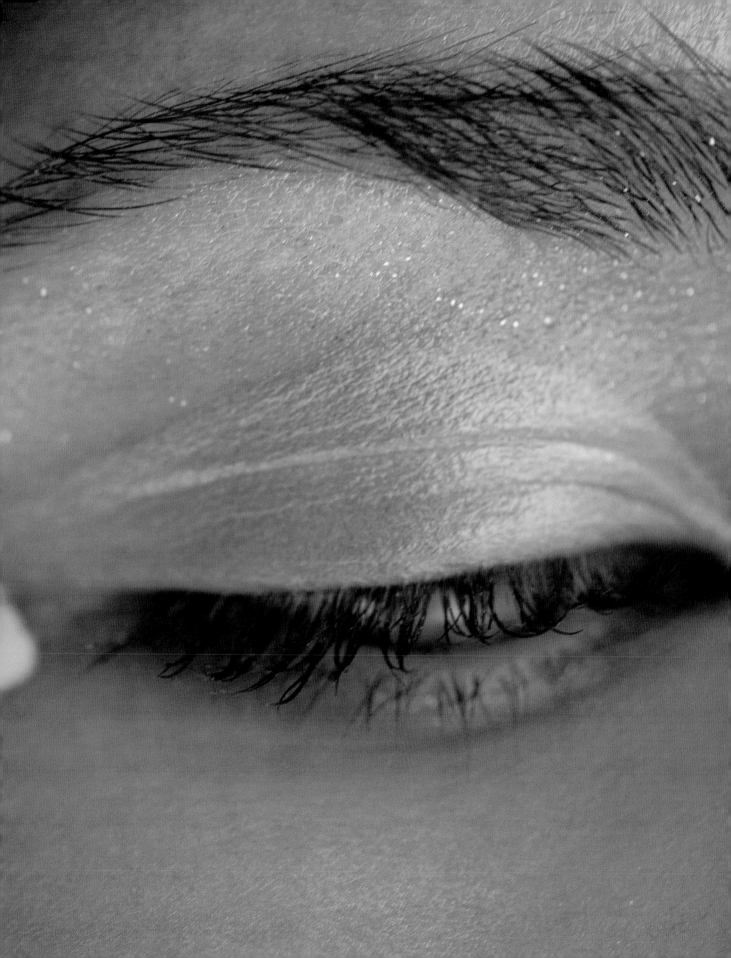

Audacious spirit. Mysterious as emeralds. Lean, mean, green sheen.

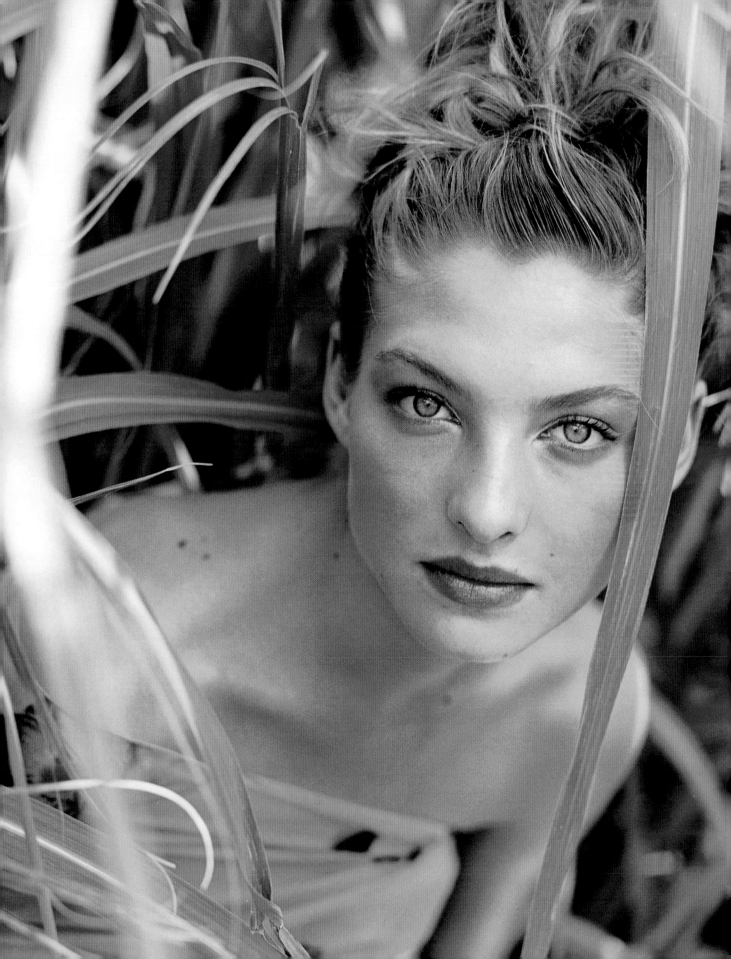

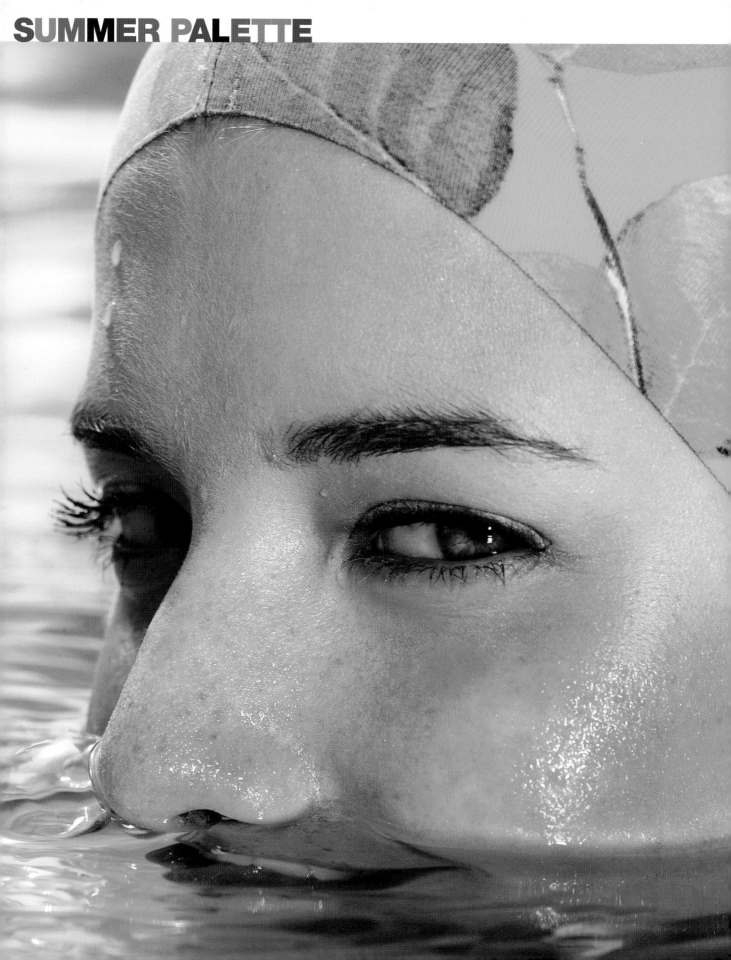

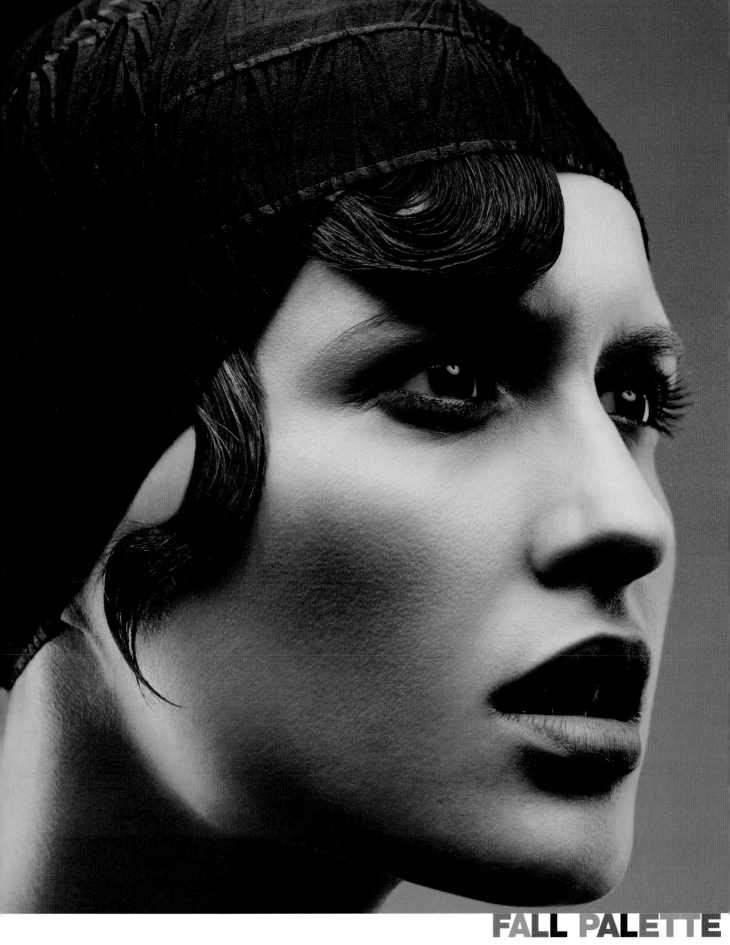

FALL PALETTE

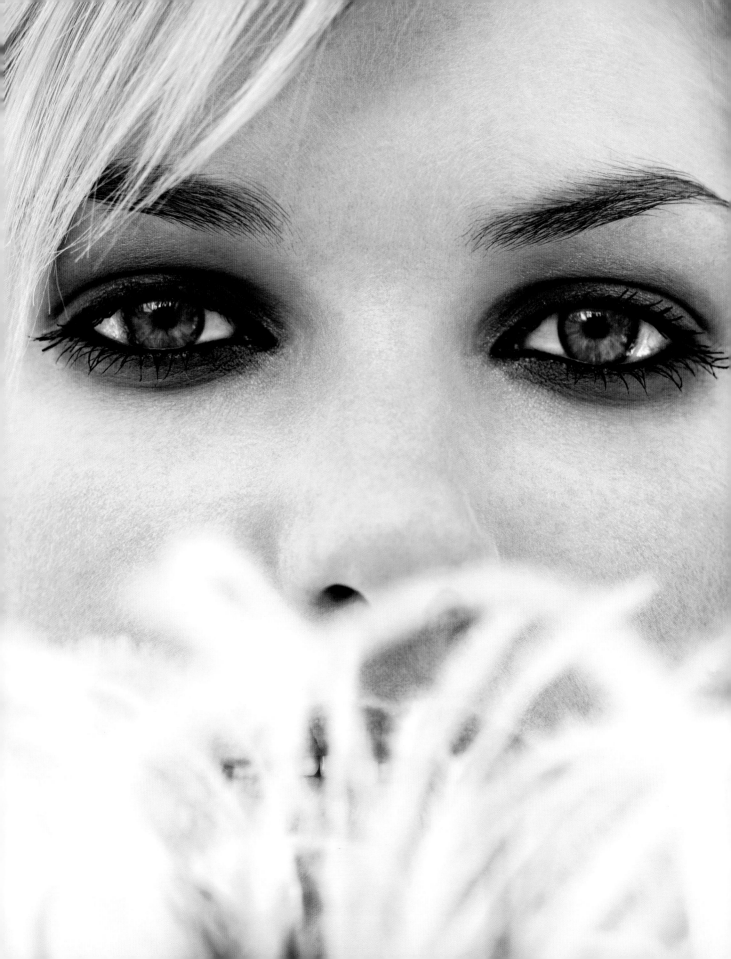

Intense gaze and frosty pallor. There's fire under the ice...

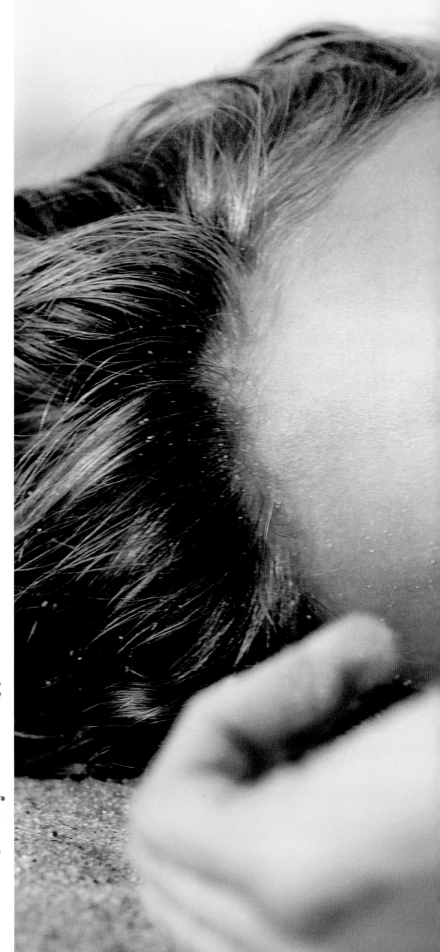

A cocktail
of
ocean blue
and marine
green
for a technicolor
siren.

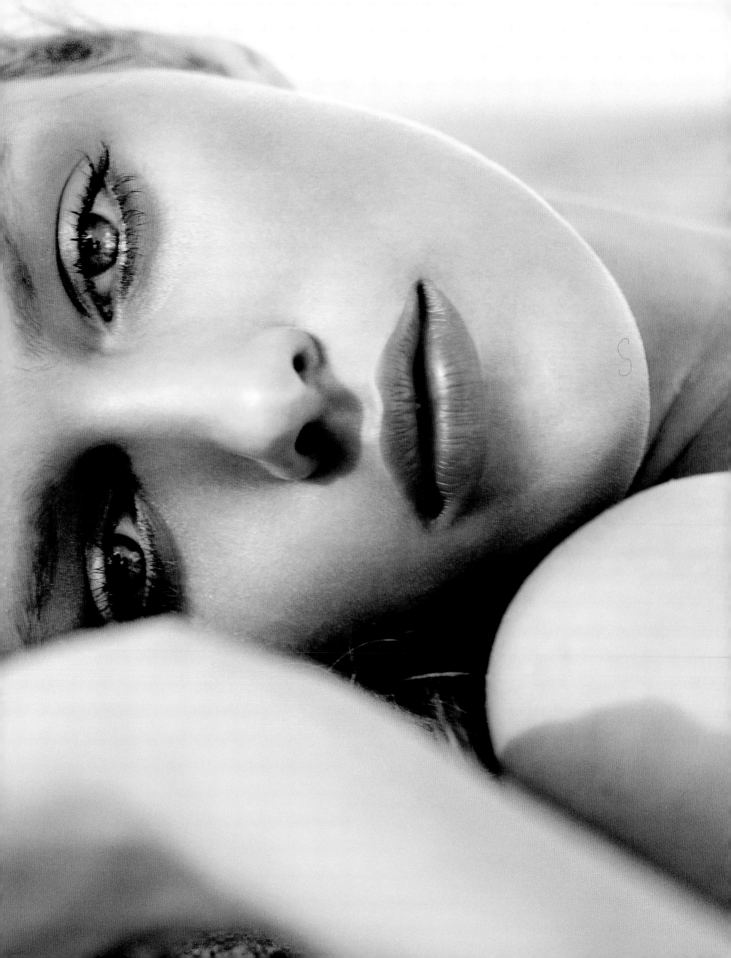

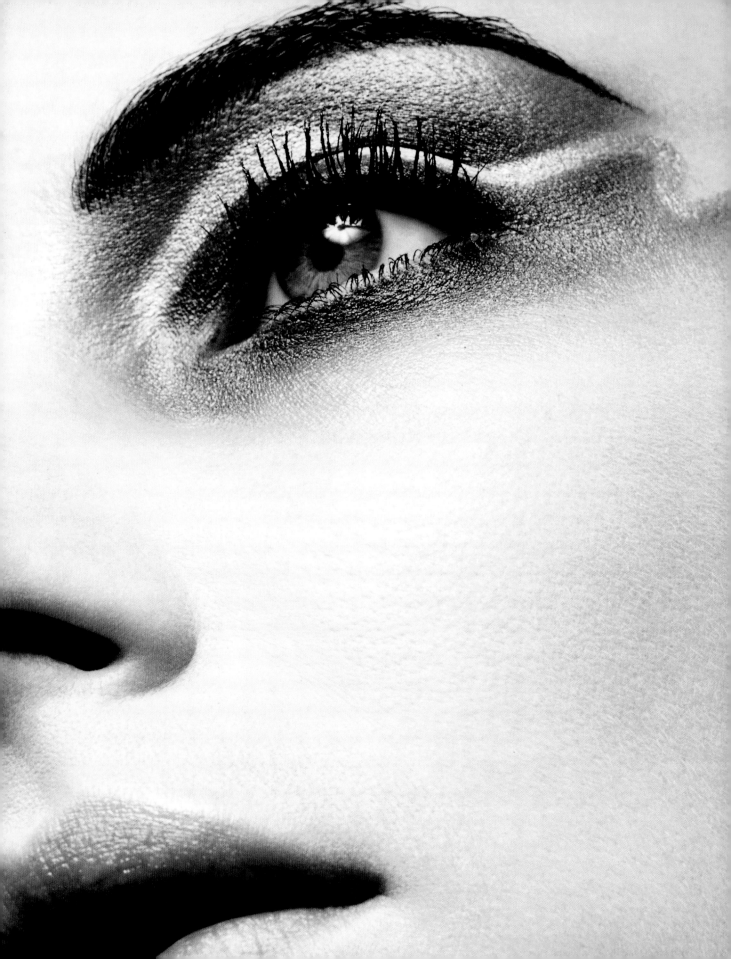

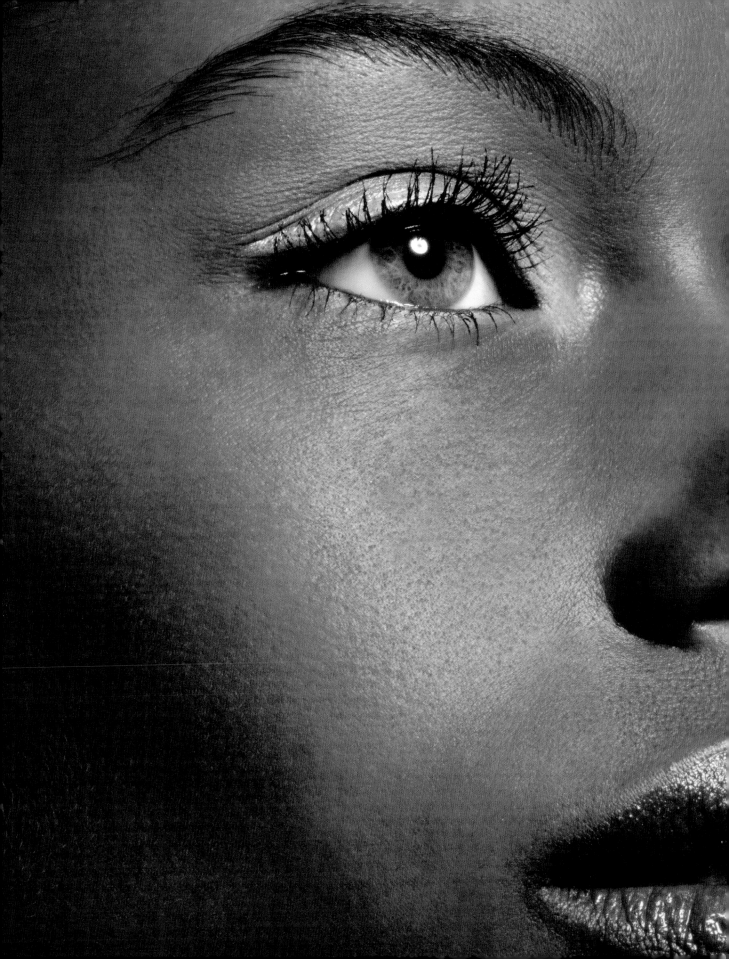

Drawing the line: smoke and smudge

The simplest of makeup accessories, there's nothing easier than a swipe of eyeliner to bring out your personality. Here are some simple tips to help you keep your eye on the ball.

TIPPING YOUR BEAUTY SCALE To find the right pencil for you, test on the back of your hand to achieve the right texture. If it is too dry, it won't leave as much color as you'd like and you could hurt yourself by having to apply too hard. On the other hand, if it's too soft, the color will undoubtedly smudge. For maximum precision, look for a soft yet firm tip that is sufficiently supple to follow your lead, depending on the desired effect: smudged or smart.

COLOR CONSCIOUS The possibilities are limitless with tints for every occasion: from matte to shimmery and from muted to pearly, eyeliner can add unbelievable depth to your eyes. Sober dark tones will add fire to blue and green irises but will bring out the gold in hazels and dark browns.

A TIP FROM TERRY (BY TERRY)

To ensure maximum hold, gently stretch and hold your eyelid closed with a finger while applying the pencil across the whole lid.

On the bottom lid a thick line just above your lashes on the lower inner eyelid that meets the top liner at the outer corner of your eyes will really make your eyes look bigger and doe-shaped.

ADVICE FROM NICOLAS DEGENNES (Givenchy):
Look like a star: after thorough makeup removal, apply a thin line on the inner eye with a black Kohl pencil before going to bed. Your eyes are already done in the morning — just use a cotton swab to repair what's run.

What you'll need
Be sure to buy a special sharpener intended only for your eye pencils. A regular pencil sharpener is poorly suited for the task and not very hygienic.

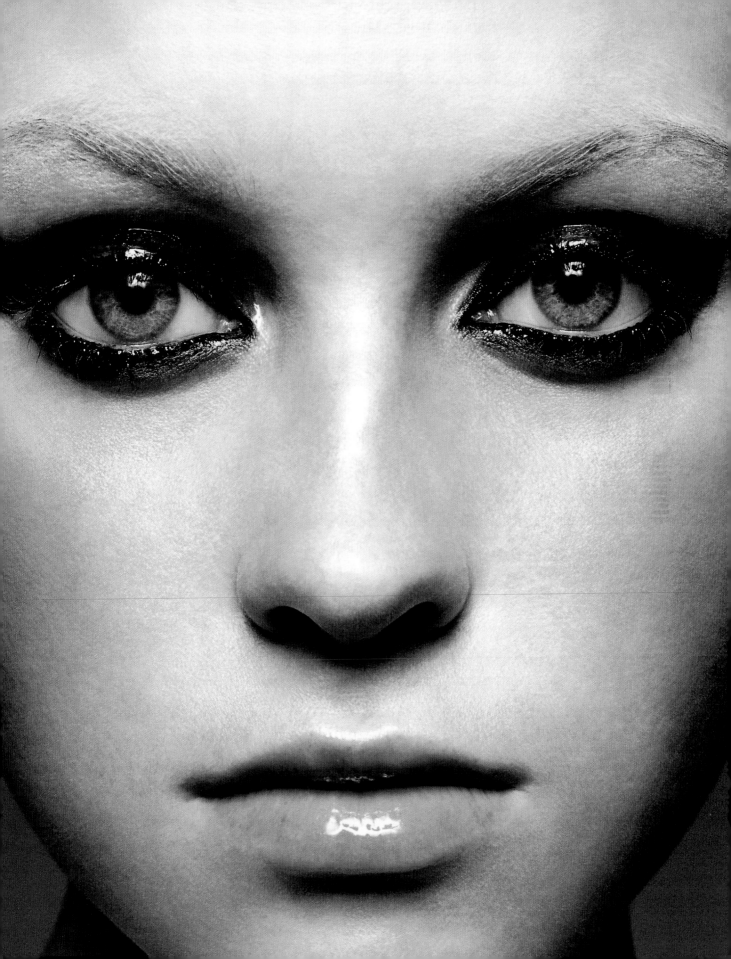

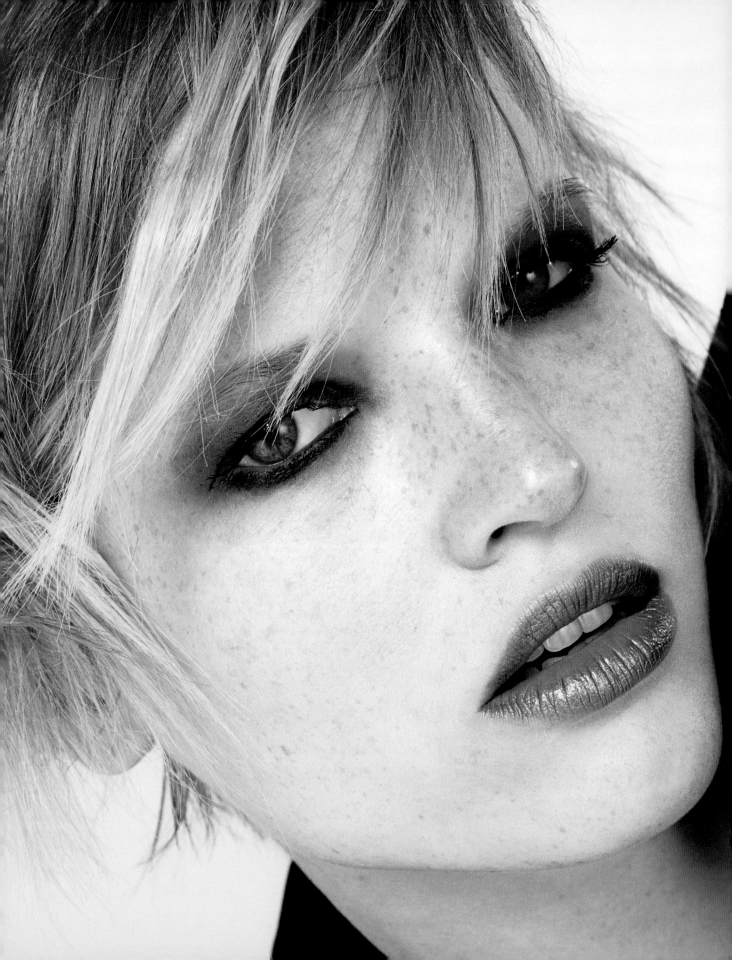

Pencil tips for looking good

Put some lead in your pencil: the art of eye definition.

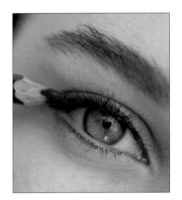

KOHL PENCILS should be warmed up first with your hand (or on a light bulb): the color effect on your lids will be even more dramatic. Apply between your lashes for greater depth. Lightly pulling on the tip of your eyelid will help draw color underneath. Smudge with a brush but beware of closing off the outer corner: it can result in a too-heavy look.

KEEPING A LID ON SHADOWS Starting from the bottom of your lashes, use a zigzag movement for blurring. To achieve a limpid look, smudge a bit with your fingertip (you can use a dot of your eye concealer) or with a pencil. Hold your eyelid while applying for maximum definition, and don't be afraid to run over a bit above: Terry says that it gives a younger look to your eyes.

TIPS & TRICKS

FANCY YOUR FLAWS

To correct eyes that are too close together use a lighter pencil from the inner corner until the middle of your eye, then finish off with a darker tone at the outer edges.

To perk up droopy eyes start with a darker color then finish off with something lighter …

ADVICE FROM TERRY (by Terry): A bright spot of light and cool mauve shadow around your eye will brighten things up and make your eyes look more rested.

In the line of sight: just one aim … and just one shot.

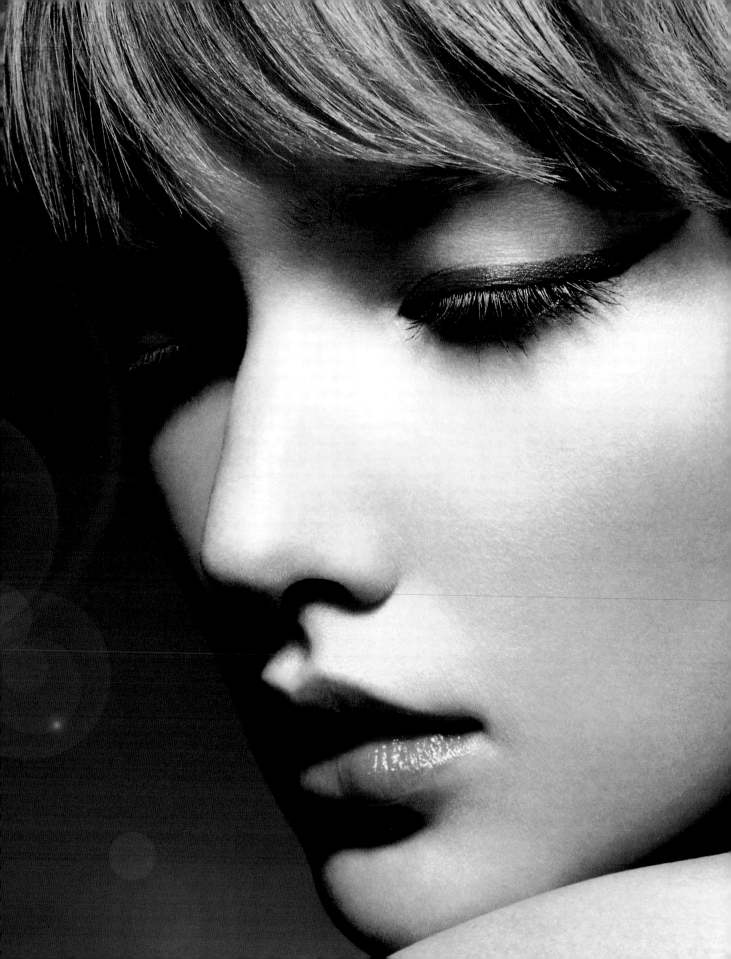

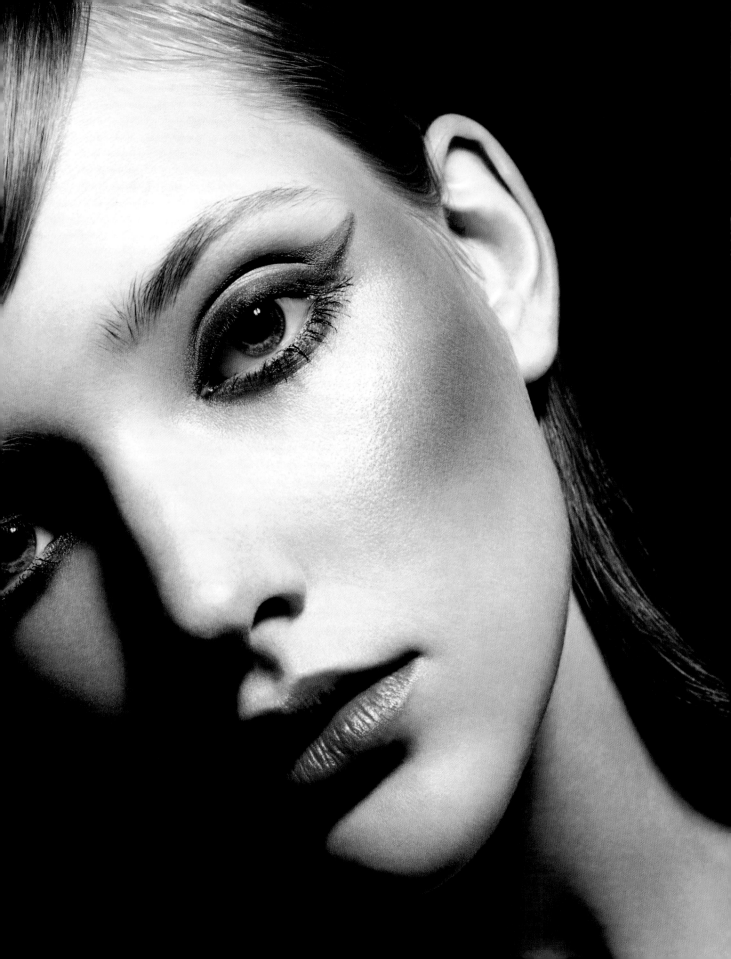

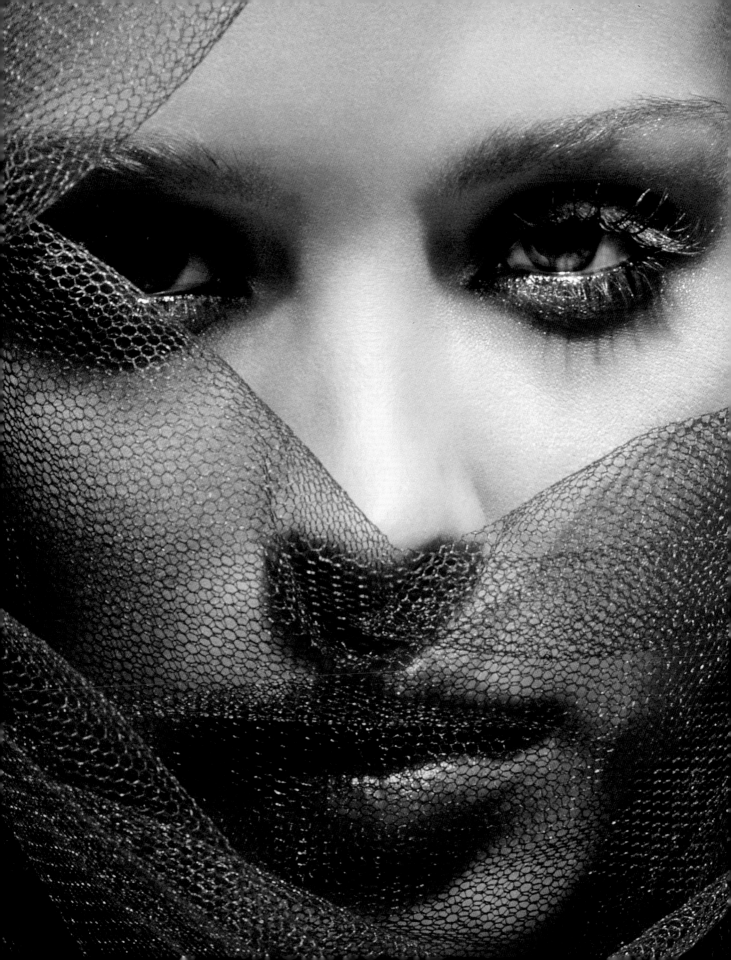

Give 'em an eyeful

It's a comeback for the makeup star of the Seventies: new liquid and gel formulas do away with brushes and invite your boldest doodles yet!

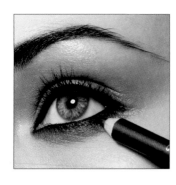

1 **DOE, A DEER ... Eyelids:** To prevent uncontrolled excess, firmly hold your lid with one finger while applying from the inner corner. Work gradually towards the middle, thickening as desired, and then finish off starting from the outer corner. Be sure that both lines are equal.

Lower lid: Same principle: start with a thin line from the inner corner and then join it with the outer with a slight upward movement.

2 **MATCHING TONES UPPER LID:** For guaranteed elegance: overlap shades of subtly smudged eye shadows with the lightest tones on top and complete the look with thin eyeliner matching your iris. **Lower lid:** A broad stroke that softly runs over into the inner eyelid will give your gaze immediate intensity.

3 **OPTICAL ILLUSIONS Enlarge your eyes** by accentuating your upper eyelid: start from the inner corner and aim for your ear. **To correct a "droopy" look**, highlight your lower lid by working away from the eyelash line as you get closer to your nose.

4 **HAUTE COUTURE** A bold choice that will also bring out your personality and your creativity: let it all hang out!

ADVICE FROM PATRICK LORENTZ (Estée Lauder) Always pick a thin and supple brush, and don't put too much liner on it: this is the best way to prevent smearing and runs.

Top stitch equals top glamour? The look in picture 4 and on the opposite page is achieved with the flat end of the brush. Keep your skin taut while applying by placing your finger just above your cheek bones and lightly pulling downwards.

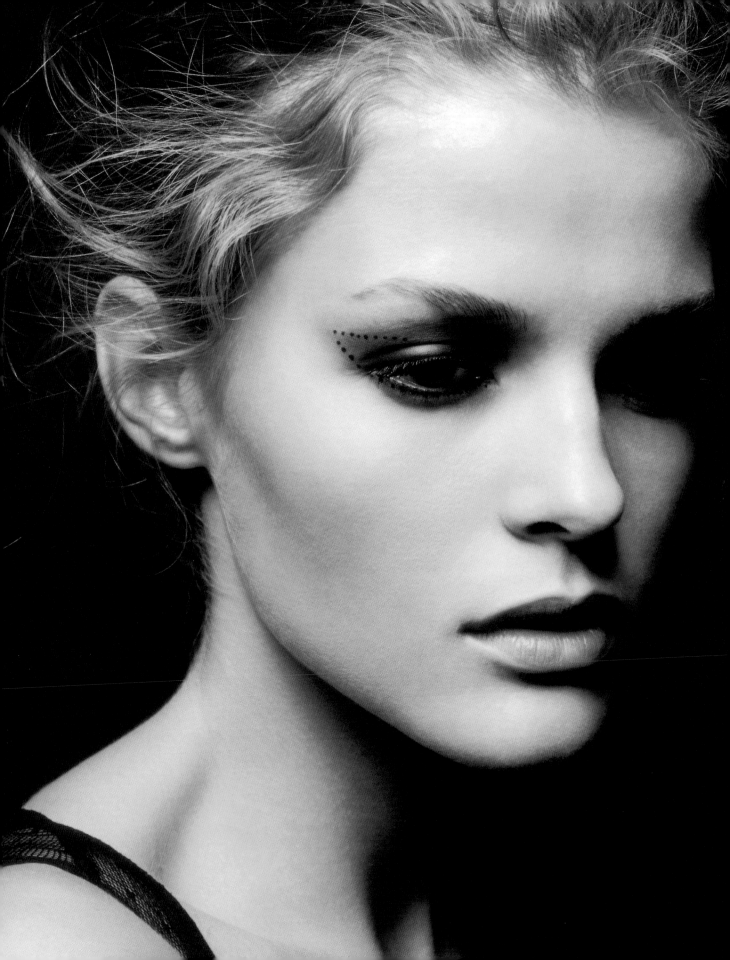

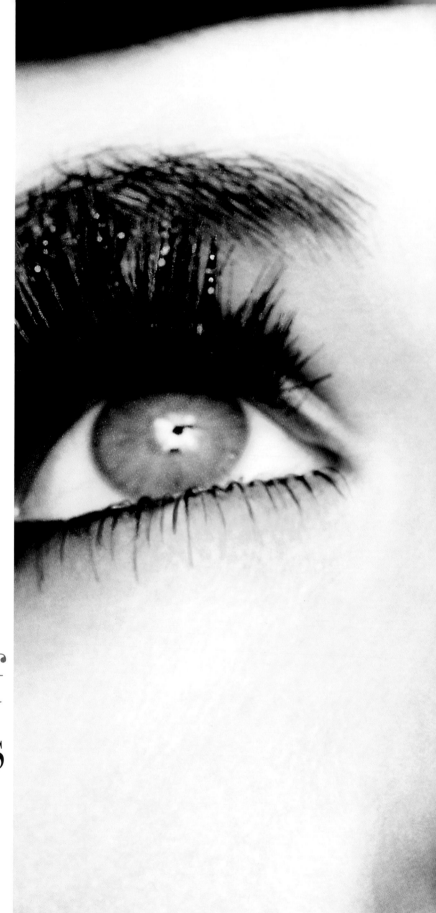

EYES: LASHES

Don't wait for tears to bead to show off your feelings

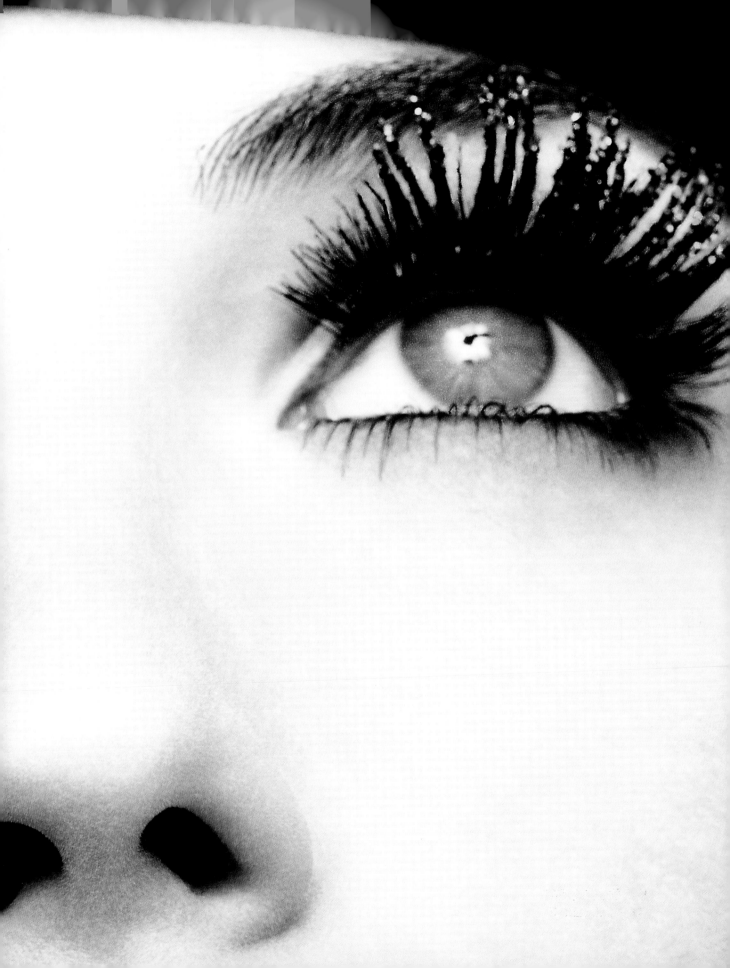

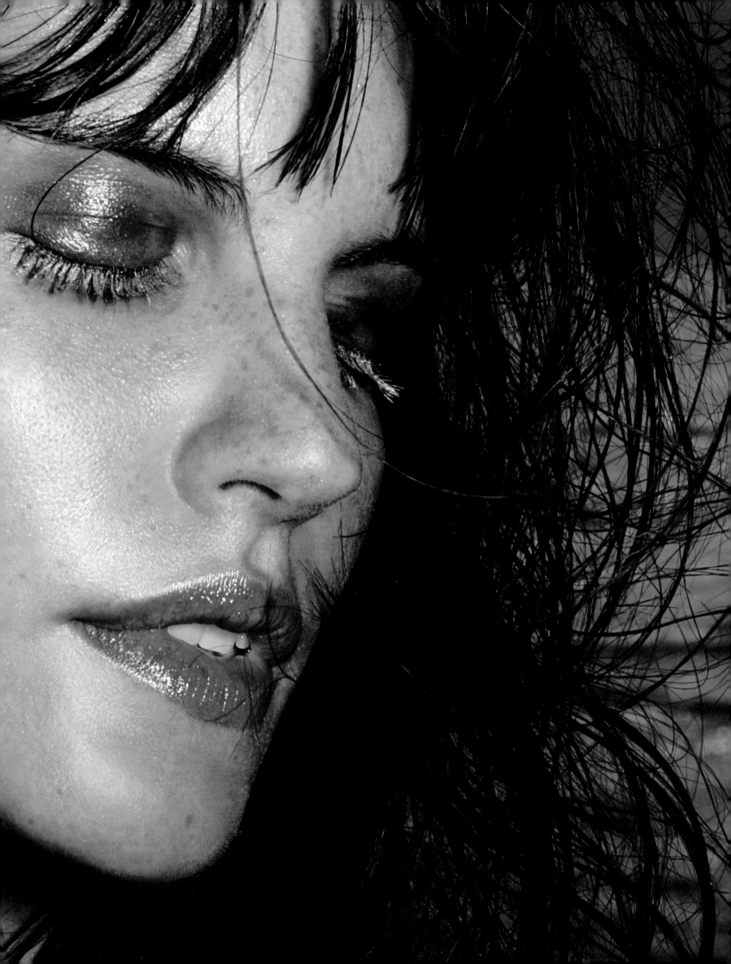

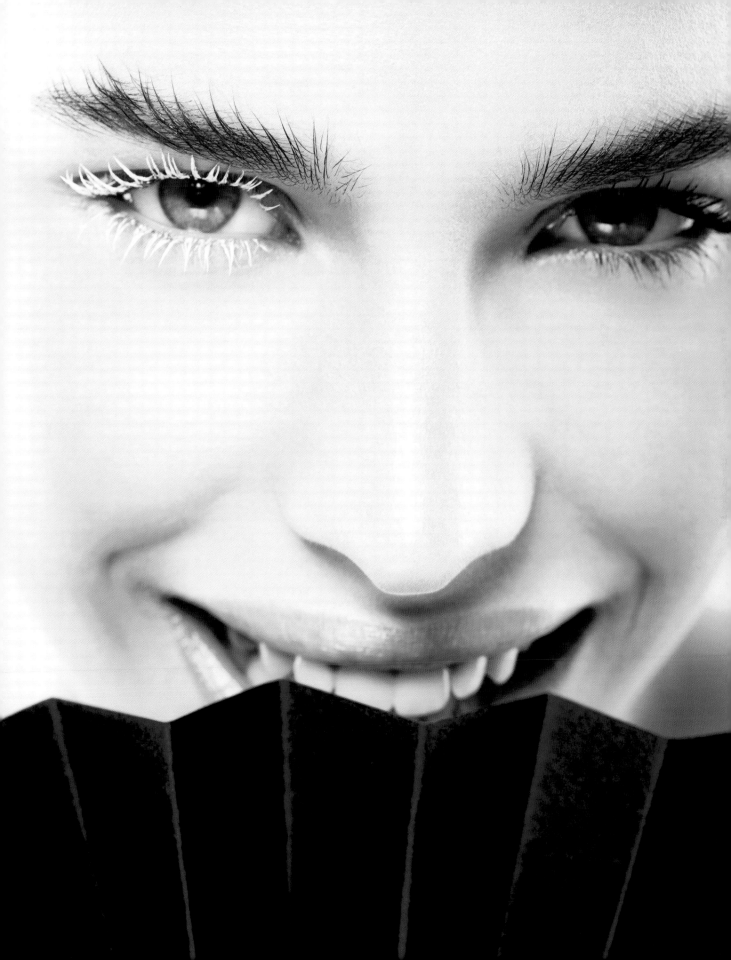

Without batting a lash

Thickened, lengthened or curled to perfection, maximize their volume for the most glamorous lashes imaginable. Mascara sets the stage for an eye-stopping show.

1 **Start from scratch** Your lashes should be spotlessly clean before getting underway. Soothe your lids with a touch of concealer.

2 **Ideal Curves** Long live eyelash curlers, they are the preferred choice of professional makeup artists. But use them only on clean lashes, otherwise you risk damaging or breaking them.

3 Here's one way to **thicken eyelashes** before applying mascara — a (very light) veil of translucent powder.

4 If your mascara is a two-step process, start with **the lash fortifier** made from cellulose fibers that lengthens and thickens while it treats your lashes.

5 Apply mascara on the top of your lashes first, then from the roots, maintaining the curve in your movement. **For maximum volume** leave the brush for a few seconds on the tips of freshly curled lashes. Start from the roots to ensure straight lashes instead of outward-pointing ones. Repeat the process until you have achieved the desired look.

ADVICE FROM IRENE OBERRAUCH (Studio makeup artist):
Make sure you close your mascara tightly so that it doesn't dry out. Contrary to what you might think, dipping the wand in and out does not ensure even distribution but only dries out the product by forcing air into the tube.

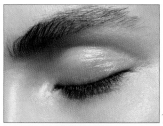

1

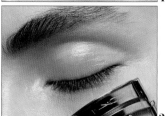

2

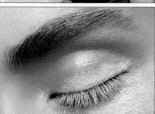

3

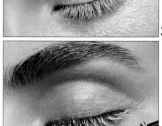

4

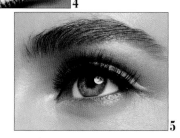

5

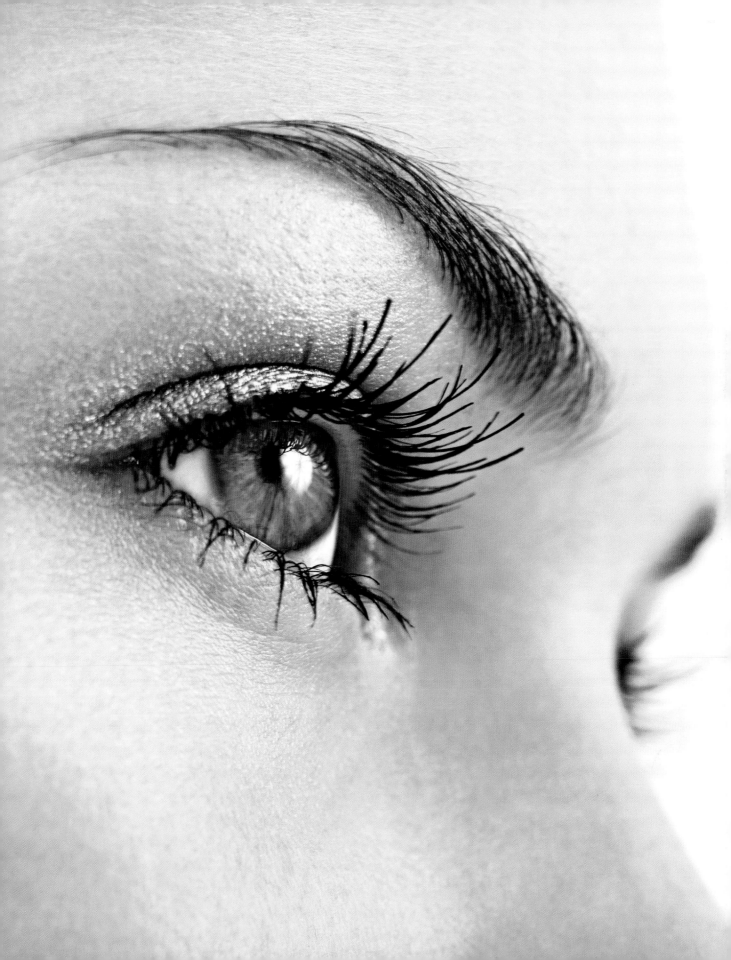

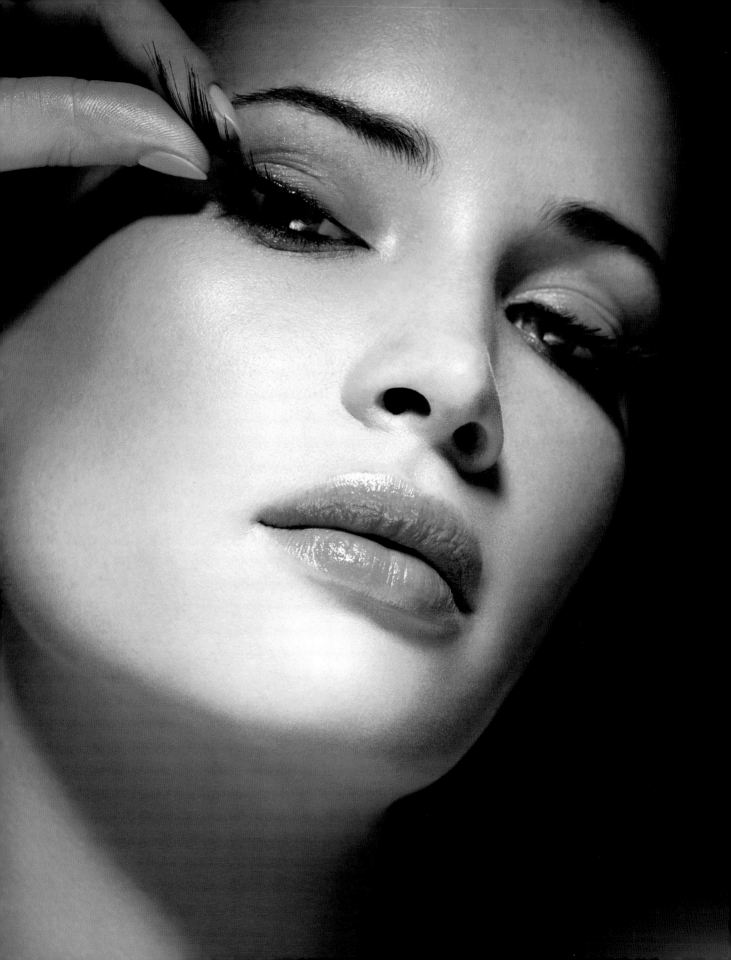

Fake is beautiful!

Perfect for the evening, you have nothing to fear: fake lashes go to great lengths to appear natural. Make a short story long!

1 To have an idea of the final result, simply place the fake lashes on top of your own: if you find them too long, don't be afraid to trim them with scissors. Keep your hand steady and cut in one snip to guarantee a pretty shape.

2 Apply a thin line of eyelash glue to the base end of the lashes (with a little more on the edges since they're more likely to unstick). Blowing on the glue for a few seconds will ensure greater hold.

3 Starting from the inner corner, place the lashes as close to your own lash line as possible.

4 While waiting for the glue to dry, gently tap with the end of a brush to perfect positioning. Do your best not to blink so that the glue sticks correctly.

5 Round off the look with a very thin line of eyeliner to blur the line where fake meets real. Mascara will guarantee as natural a look as possible.

ADVICE FROM LOUISE WITTLICH (Studio makeup artist)
Take your time. Finish one eye before starting the second.

How do I take them off?
Unstick them carefully, starting at the outer edge. Any remaining glue can easily be removed with sweet almond oil.

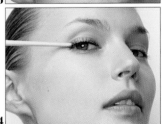

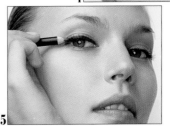

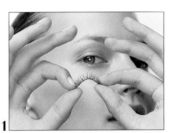

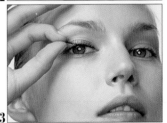

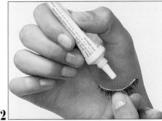

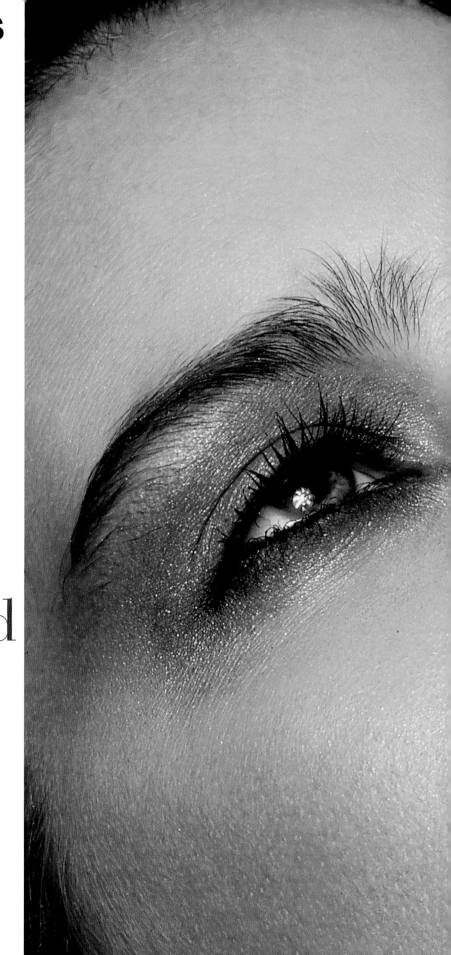

Powders and shadow perfectly blended for the liveliest of canvases.

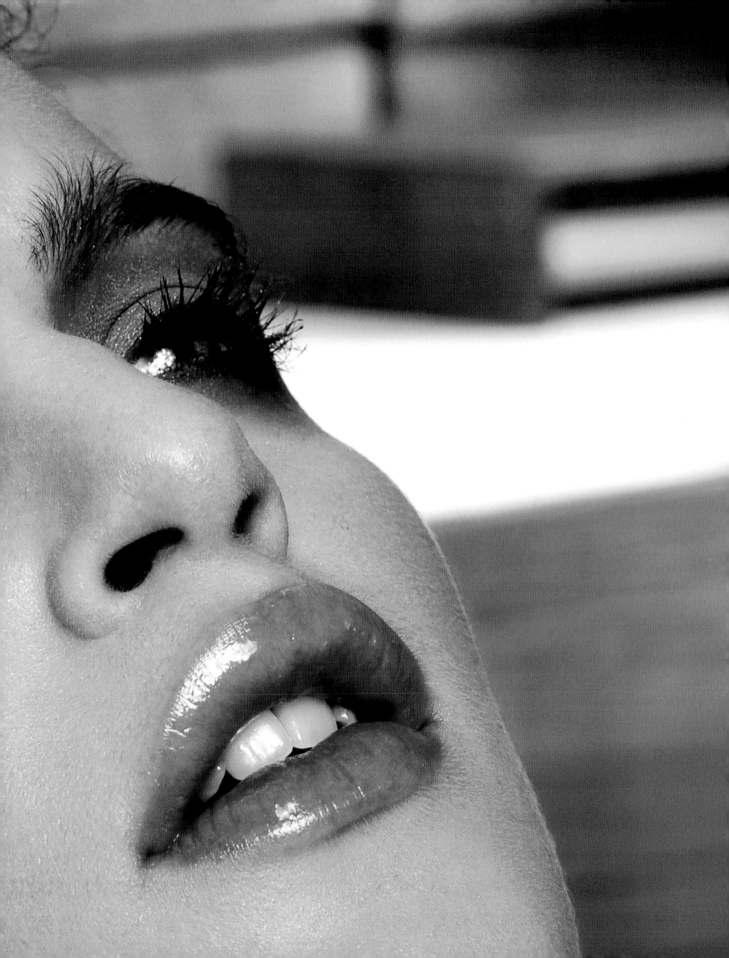

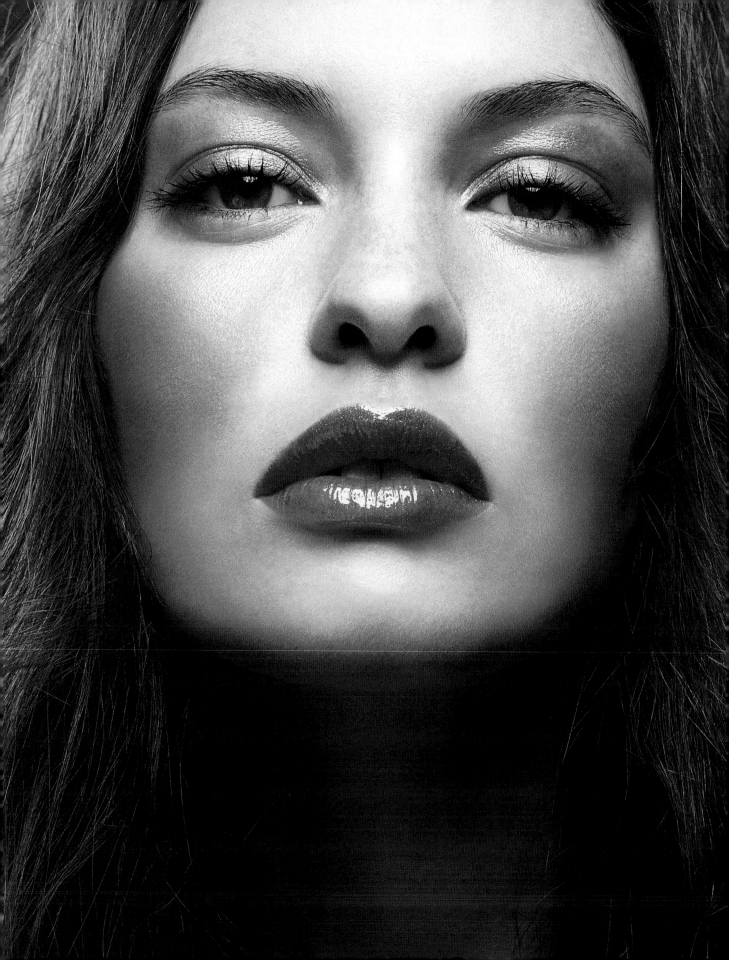

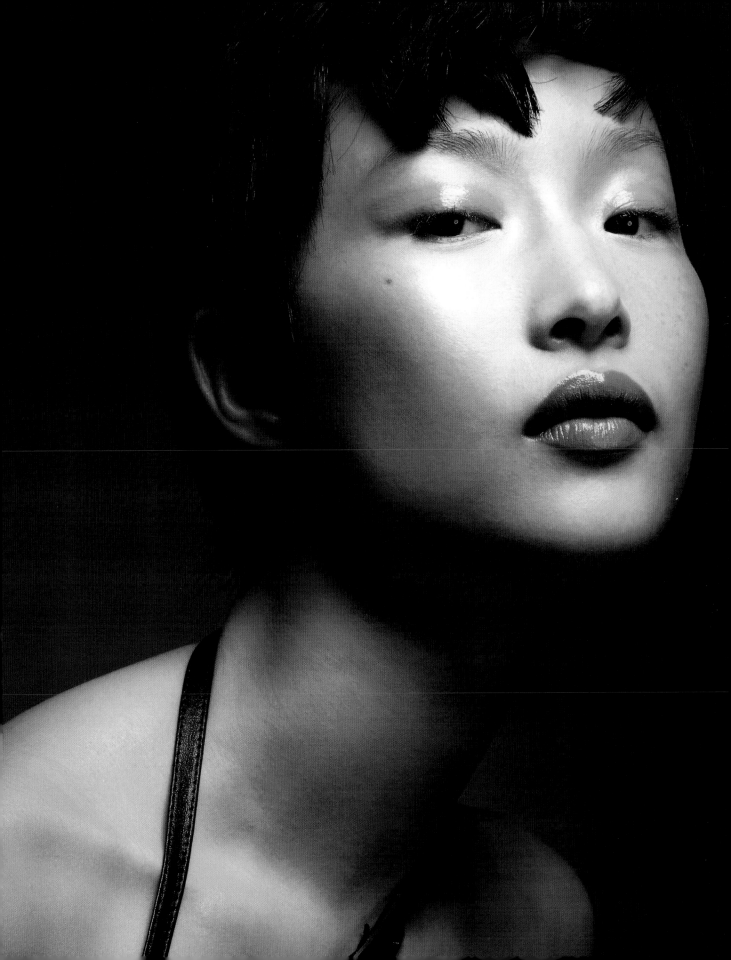

Where there's smoke, there's fire

It's a paradox: "smoky" tones bring light to your look. With a skilled hand, prunes become the new apple of your eye!

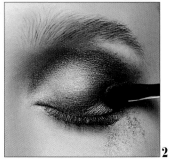

1 **TO WIDEN YOUR EYES** Use a lighter shade in the inner corner and fan outwards with a darker one. If you're going for transparency, a brush is your best bet.

2 **FOR A MORE INTENSE LOOK,** just like on the outer edge of the eyelid, use a dampened sponge-brush dipped in shadow to blend for longer wear and more intense color.

BIGGER ... A small touch of iridescent powder on the corner of your eyelids will make them look larger, as well as a lighter shade dusted on your brow bones just under the eyebrows.

DEEPER ... Running slightly over the outside edges will make them look less narrow. A halo effect around the arch (see photo at right) will also give depth.

A line of prune kohl pencil is a perfect finish for an elegant evening look.

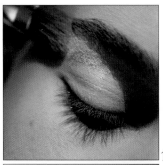

ADVICE FROM SUZANNE STERLING (Chanel)
I recommend a flat, square-tipped brush for eye shadow application. You can smudge with a rounded brush after. To magnify your eyes: a small touch of a brighter powder smack in the middle of the upper lid.

What you'll need
• square brush
• round brush
• prune-colored eye shadow
• light-iridescent eye shadow

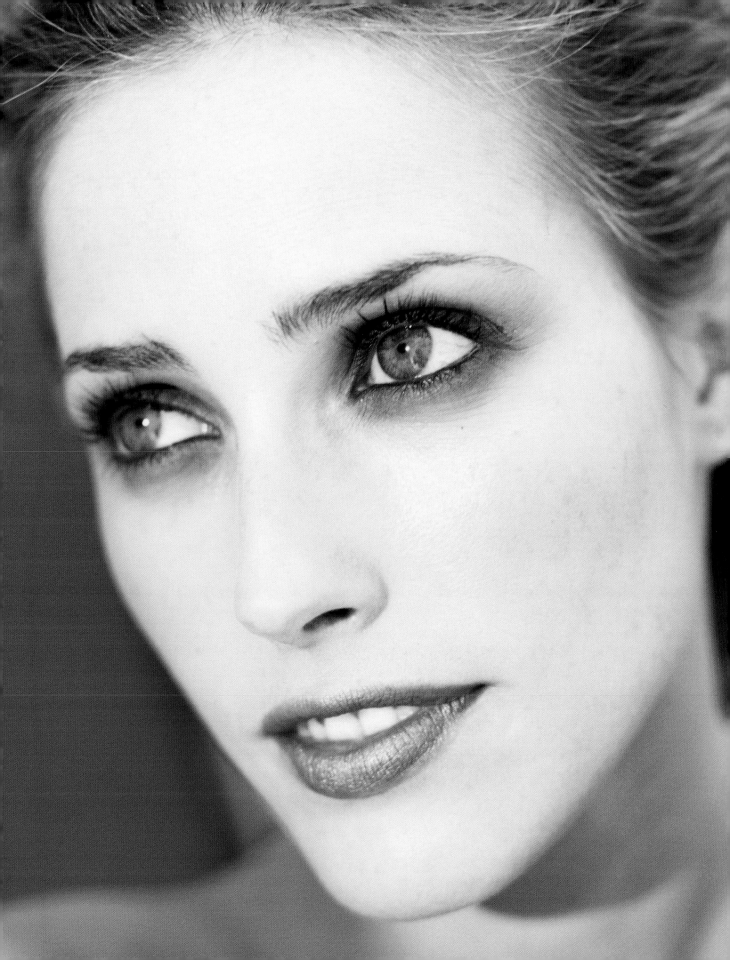

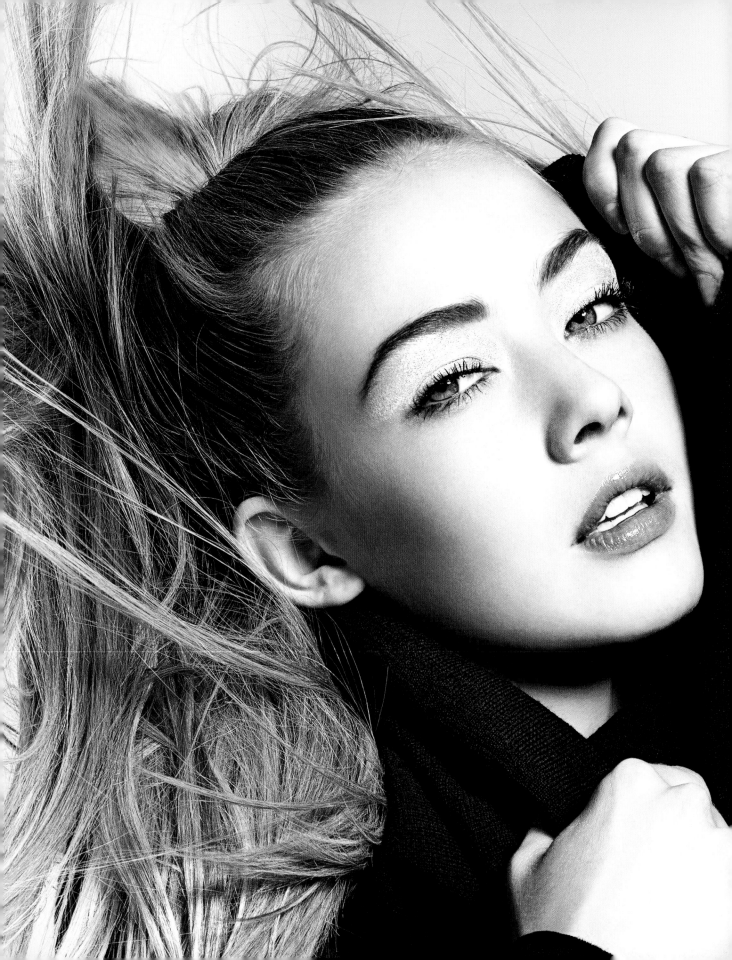

Metallic magic

Straight from the goldsmith: golden drops and silver powders are refined but not too flashy. Let the party begin!

1 Eyelash curlers Again, use only on clean lashes and start at the roots. Curlers will prevent you from overdoing it with mascara.

2 Concealer Blend it in under your eye, from the inner to the outer corners, following the lash line.

3 Use a brush to apply the first coppery coat at the base of your eyelid, starting from the inside corner and then under your lower lashes. Add a silvery note and blend upwards towards your eyebrows.

4 Sketch a pearly V on the inner corner of your eye to give **a touch of light.**

5 Keeping your eyelid taut, **drawn a thin line of eyeliner** from the inside working your way out, and finish off with a coat of mascara.

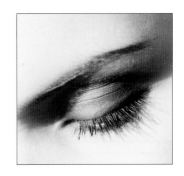

ADVICE FROM JAMES KALIARDOS (L'Oréal Paris): Opt for a kohl pencil if you are weary of liquid eyeliner.

What you'll need
- eyelash curler
- narrow brush
- thick eyeshadow brush
- concealer
- copper shadow
- silver shadow
- eyeliner

Iridescent irises

Pink diamond and plum pearl: an irresistible pairing that will light up any pair of eyes.

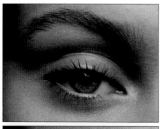
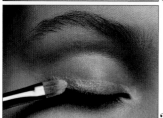
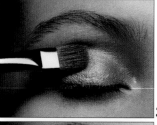
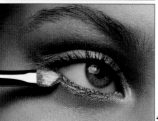

1 With your eyebrows flawlessly brushed and your lashes curled with the help of your eyelash curler, leave your lid bare: cream eyeshadow stays perfectly in place.

2 Your eye closed, place the entire amount of creamy pink shadow on the lid, spreading and blending from the lash line with a flat brush.

3 Using a larger, clean brush, blend upwards towards your brow bone to achieve total transparency.

4 While looking up, draw a line of plum shadow under your eye, working out from the inner corner.

5 For an even more sophisticated effect, smudge a bit with your finger, in the direction of your temple, before putting on mascara.

ADVICE FROM JULIE NOZIERS (Studio makeup artist):
If the result is too sparkly, use some translucent powder to tone it down. And for perfect hold, only apply powder around your eyes after you have completely finished applying your makeup.

What you'll need
- eyelash curler
- small and narrow eyeshadow brush
- full eyeshadow brush
- pink cream eyeshadow
- mauve cream eyeshadow

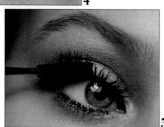

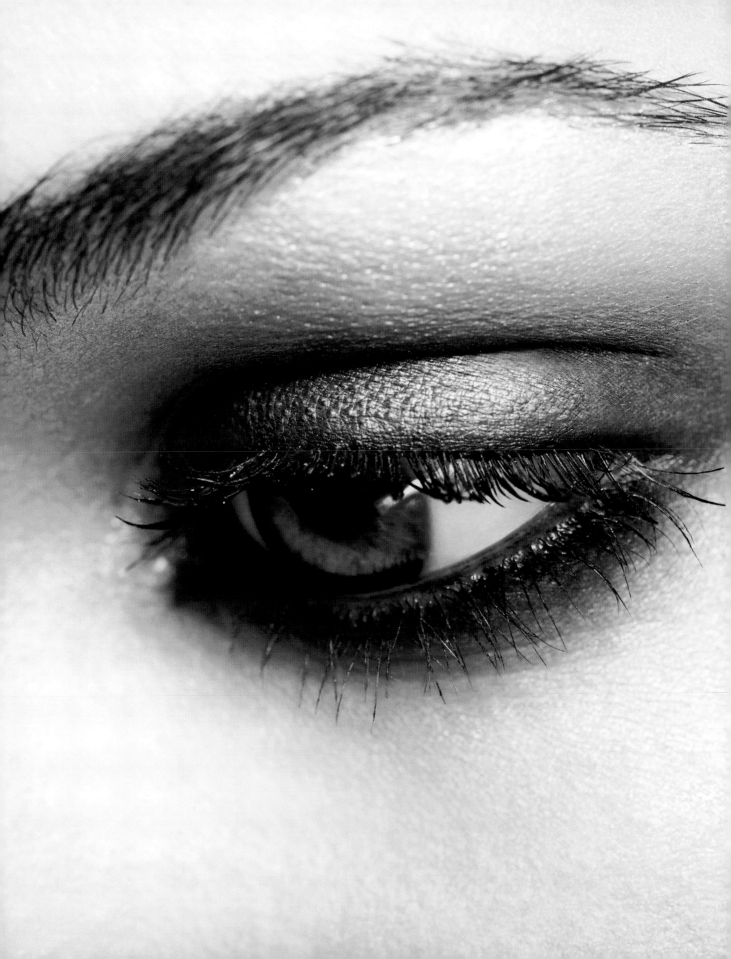

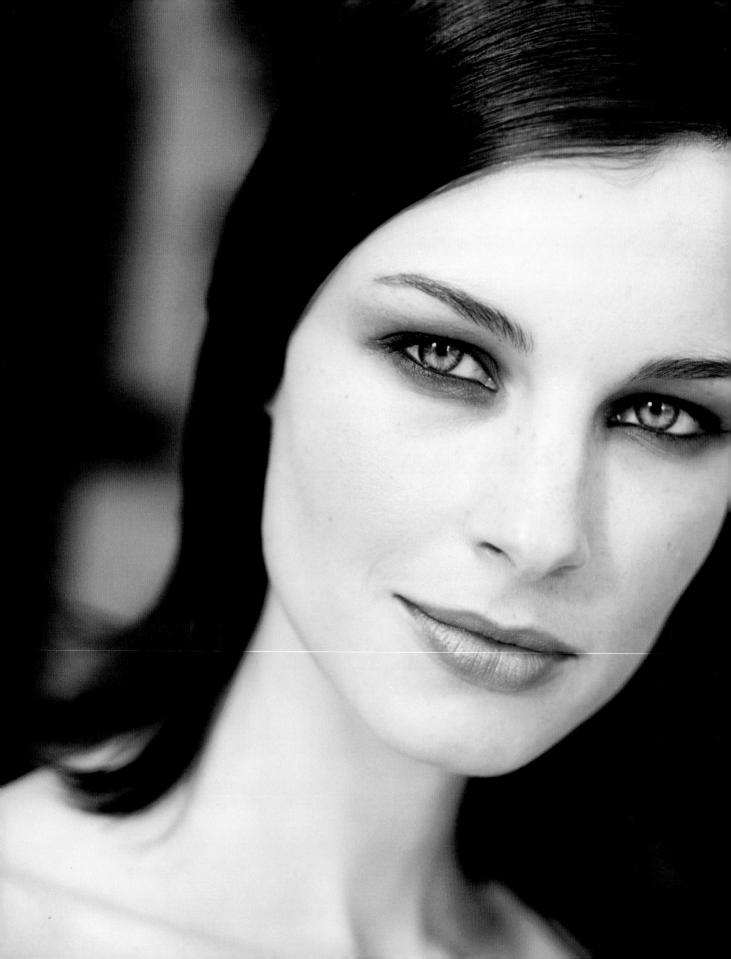

Velvety sweetness

A powdery setting for your eyes that will bring out the light in your gaze and give it depth and mystery: a velvety, matte gray will do the trick.

APPLIED WITH YOUR FINGERS, as Olivier Echaudemaison recommends for this product, smoky shades of this creamy eyeshadow will yield magnificent color gradation.

They **adapt** according to your desired intensity at any minute of the day or night. Microscopic pigments give rise to colors that are both intense and transparent for a very flattering hue. You can apply a darker tone on the entire eyelid and then blend before overlaying a lighter shade.

FOR EVENINGS, you can bring the color up to your brow bones, highlighting and creating a halo effect mirrored under your eyes.

For this look, go easy on the mascara since it is not really necessary: **opt for length rather than volume.**

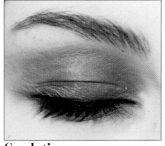

Gradation
Soft, blurred effect over the whole lid brightens up the under-eyebrow arch.

ADVICE FROM OLIVIER ECHAUDEMAISON (Guerlain):
An elegant alternative to black, which can end up too harsh, smoky grays give you a refined ashy look that intensifies dark eyes or adds limpidity and depth to lighter eyes.

What you'll need
- smoky gray cream eyeshadow
- lengthening mascara

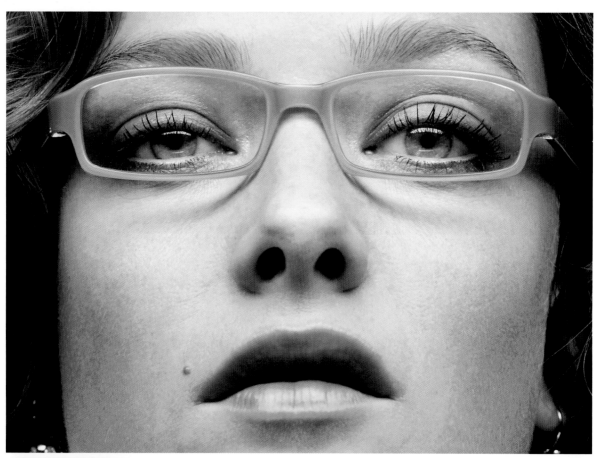
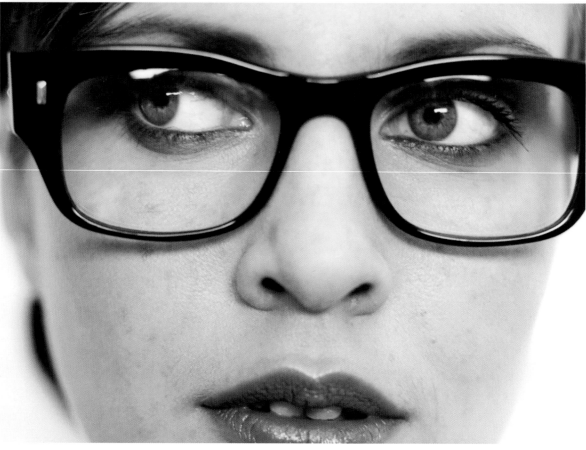

Close-up on glasses

Do you wear corrective frames? They can definitely be a beauty plus ... as long as you maintain the intensity of your gaze and master the subtle effects of makeup.

GLASSES: OPT FOR FULLY-TREATED GLASS LENSES

Regardless of the shape of your glasses, the one basic rule is to choose an anti-reflective coating for your lenses (such as Crizal Alisé Essilor) that will keep the splendor of your eyes intact. It will only take one try with an untreated lens to see that all your makeup efforts are for naught!

IF YOU ARE NEARSIGHTED your glasses might have a tendency to make your eyes look smaller. Reinforce your features with eyeliner and use extra mascara as well.

IF YOU ARE FARSIGHTED OR PRESBYOPIC, your eyes will look larger through your glasses. Definitely flattering but the magnifying effect is ruthless. James Kaliardos recommends taking great care in choosing brushes and mascara in order to have well-separated eyelashes and prevent any unattractive build-up. For the same reason, eye shadow must also be blended with great care.

ADVICE FROM JAMES KALIARDOS (L'Oréal Paris)
Choose your brushes according to how you plan on using them and clean them regularly, especially since your eyes are far more sensitive and prone to allergies than other areas of your face.

Touch-up work:
To makeup for mistakes in eyeliner or mascara application, erase the slip-up with a cotton swab dipped in concealer. Next, dip the same swab in loose powder and apply to the area that needs to be redone.

You're the
star
of the **show**.

Pretty as a
picture,

you
set the **stage:**

the **frame**
comes first.

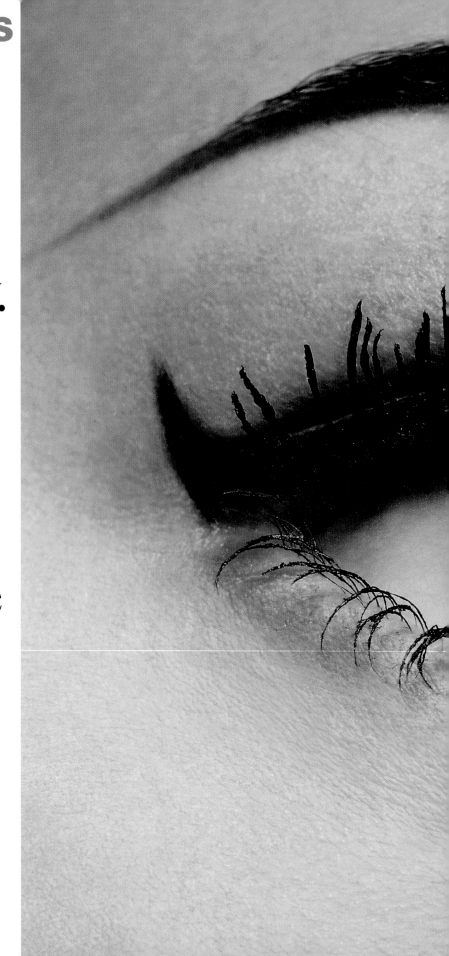

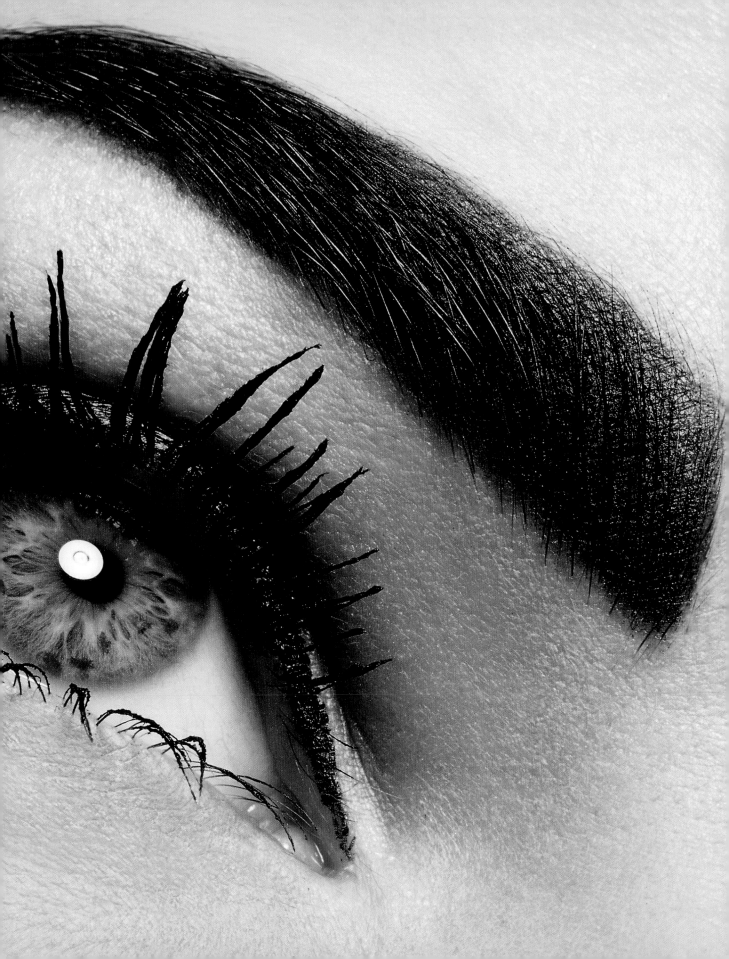

Staying in shape

Straight, arched, comma-shaped or circumflex … The shape of your eyebrows is a defining factor of your look. Treat them kindly: they are one of the first things people will notice and they say a lot about you!

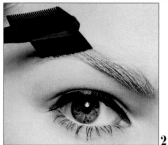

1

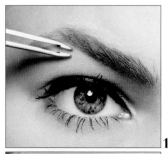

2

TWEEZING AT HOME: Comb your eyebrows first in the opposite direction of growth and then straighten them by combing the other way. Pull your skin taut using your thumb and index finger and tweeze in direction of growth. Only pluck eyebrows on the underside and thin out the brow as you work outwards. The middle should remain thick. Keep an eye on your brows in order to keep the arch clearly defined with occasional touch-ups.

TROMPE L'OEIL TECHNIQUES FOR A BALANCED FACE: If your eyes are too close together, maintain full brows from the inner corner of your eye to the arch.

To look younger: Keep your brows short with a shape that stops before the edge of your eye: low-reaching eyebrows make for a sad face. A well-defined eyebrow shape gives energy to your expression. Raising the line energizes your face and helps avoid a neglected appearance.

PENCIL TIPS Once you've combed your eyebrows into place, your brow pencil, chosen in the same shade as your eyebrows (or one shade lighter, but never darker!) will help you thicken and correct minor tweezing errors through short, thin lines, drawn in the direction of growth. Always use upward movements and work outwards from the inner corner of your eye. Blend it all together with a cotton swab.

ADVICE FROM NICOLAS DEGENNES (Givenchy)
I would suggest opting for a pencil rather than a shadow — which results in too "harsh" a look — to highlight the top of your eyebrows, and never the underside.

The right length: eyebrows should run from the inner to the outer corners of your eyes, in line with the base of your nose. It may be advisable to start off with professional brow shaping and then keep up the form with occasional plucking at home.

What you'll need
• eyebrow tweezers
• eyebrow comb
• sharp-tipped eyebrow pencil

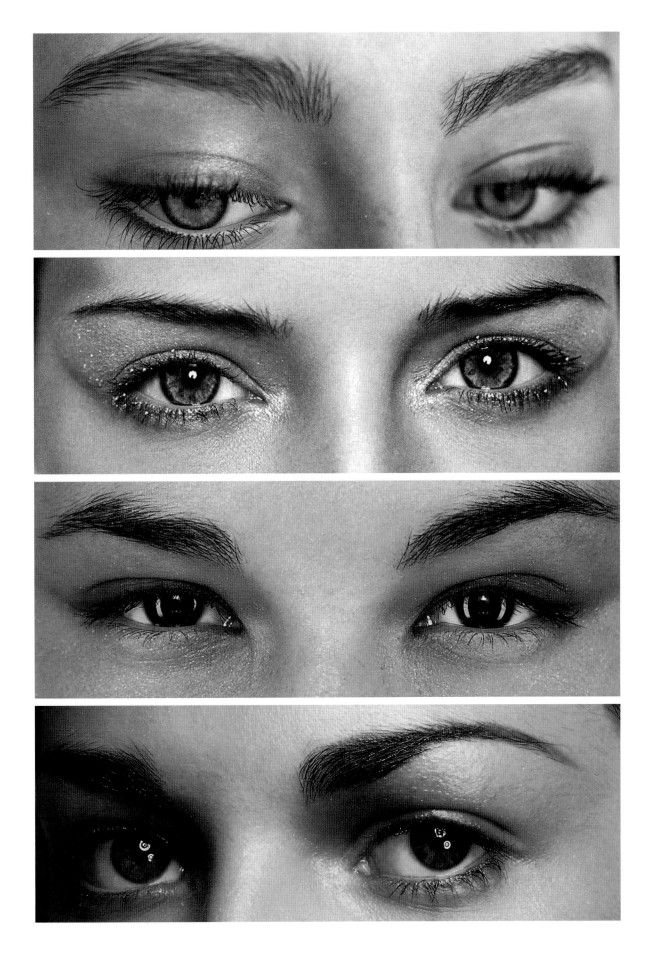

Brooke or Audrey... starry eyes

It's amazing how a little doting on your eyebrows can totally change your look. They frame your eyes: do not overlook these precious allies!

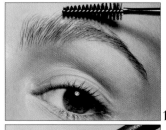

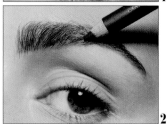

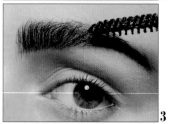

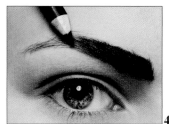

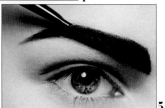

1 **A LA BROOKE SHIELDS (Tom Pecheux, Shiseido):** Your face's "coat hangers" should be straightened by upward combing without breaking the line in order to give an impression of greater width.

2 **Fill in with a pencil** (black to dark brown for dark-haired women; grey to light brown for blondes) using short, feathery strokes, starting along the underside.

3 **Blend in using an eyebrow wand,** then with a coat of mascara which will also maximize volume.

4 **A LA AUDREY HEPBURN (Terry, By Terry):** For an intensely sculpted brow: fill in eyebrows with a pencil in a robust shade that goes with your hair working outward from your nose.

5 **Even out with a brush** while drawing a well-groomed line tapering elegantly at the ends. The brush will fill in the natural shape of your eyebrows while distributing color. Use dry beauty oil or transparent mascara for the final touch.

What you'll need
- professional eyebrow tweezers
- eyebrow comb
- beveled-edge eyebrow brush
- eyebrow wand
- eyebrow pencil
- clear eyebrow mascara

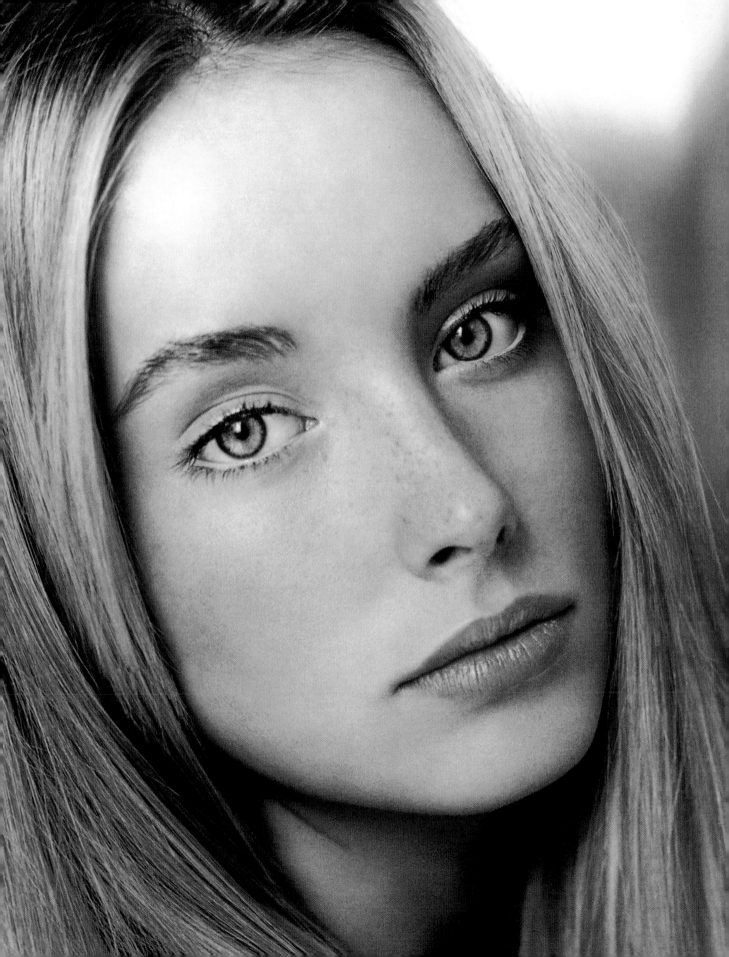

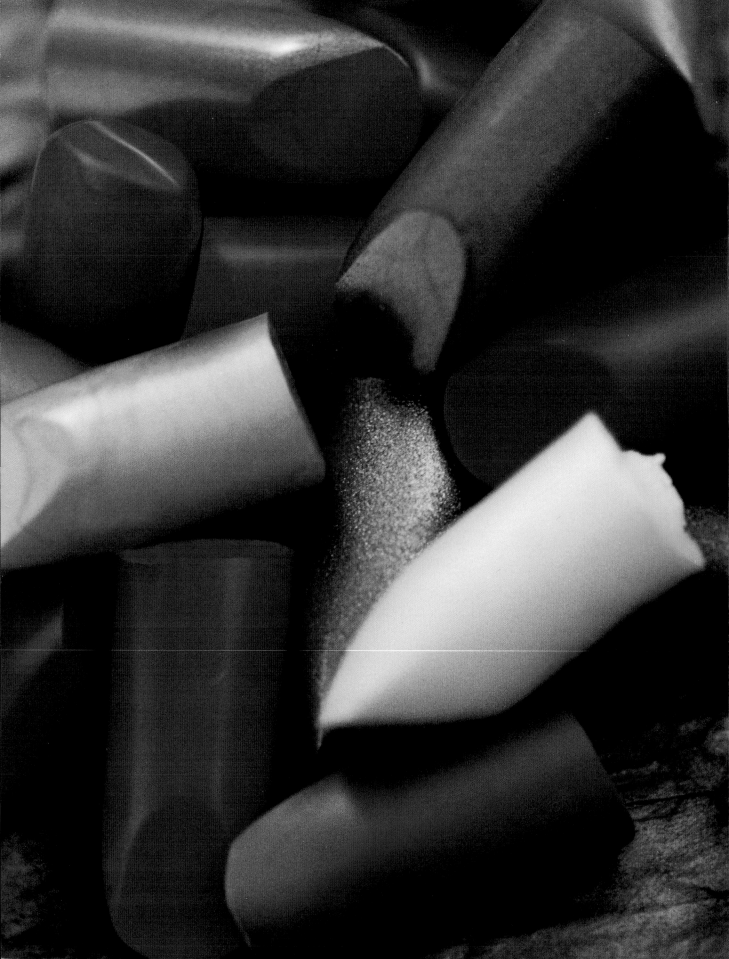

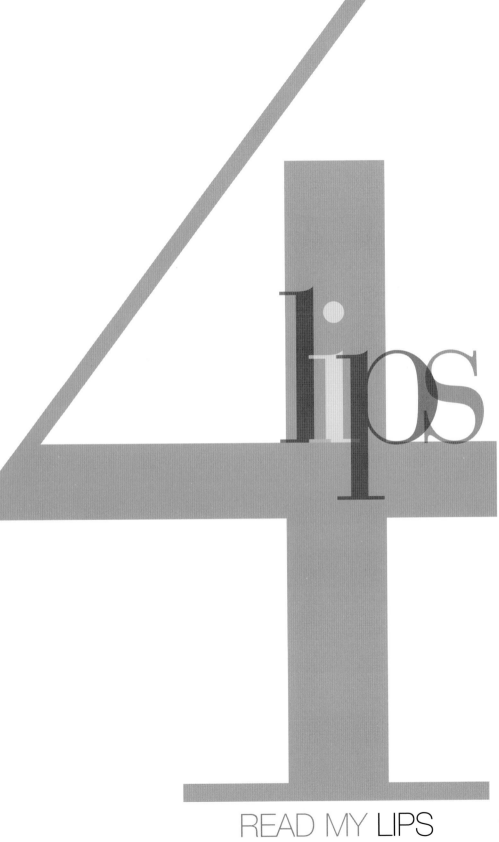

4 lips

READ MY LIPS

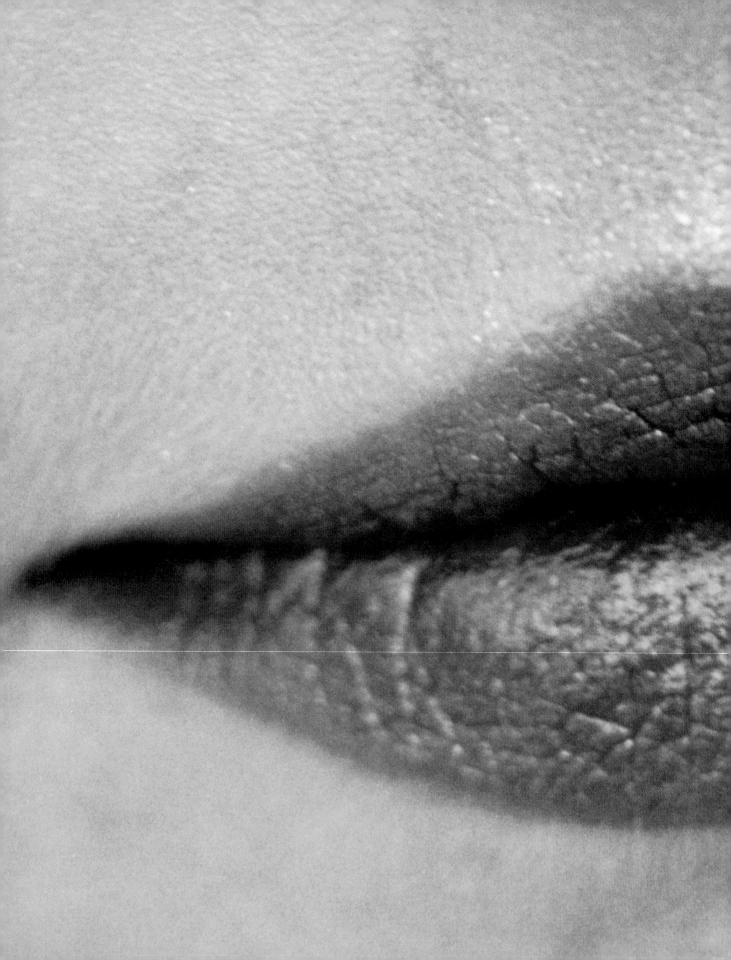

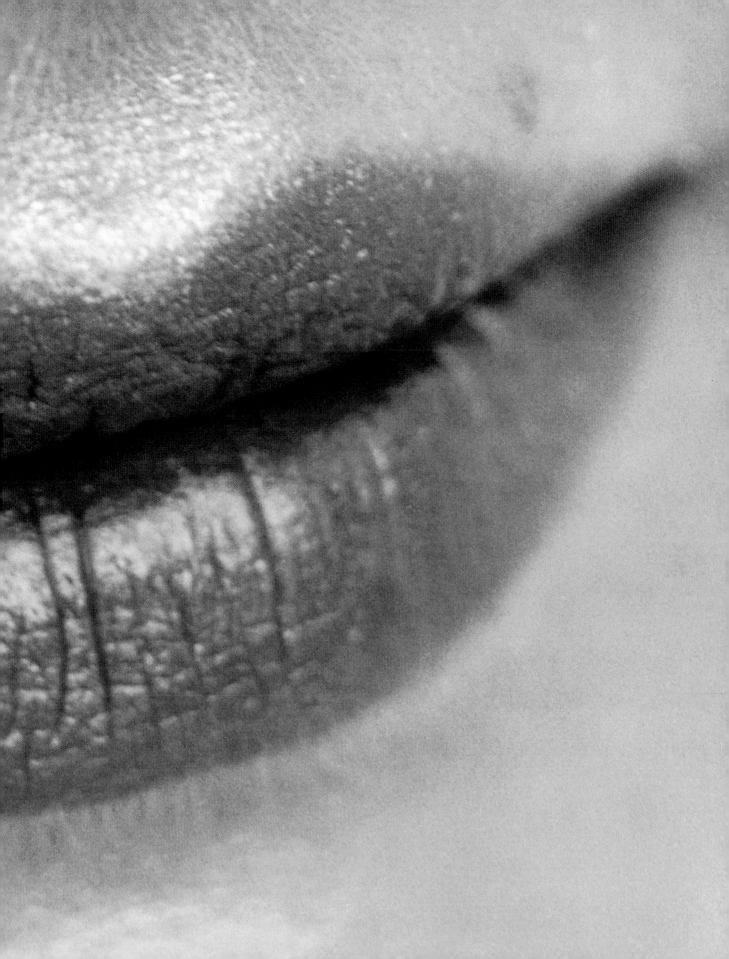

Fresh and natural, perfectly pink. Pucker up!

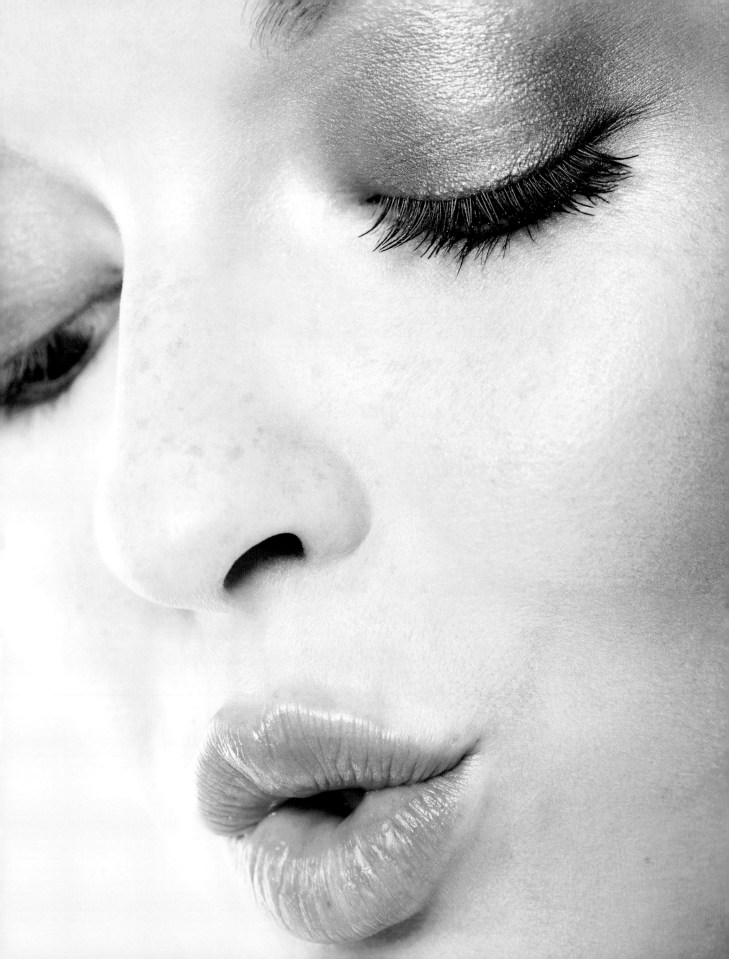

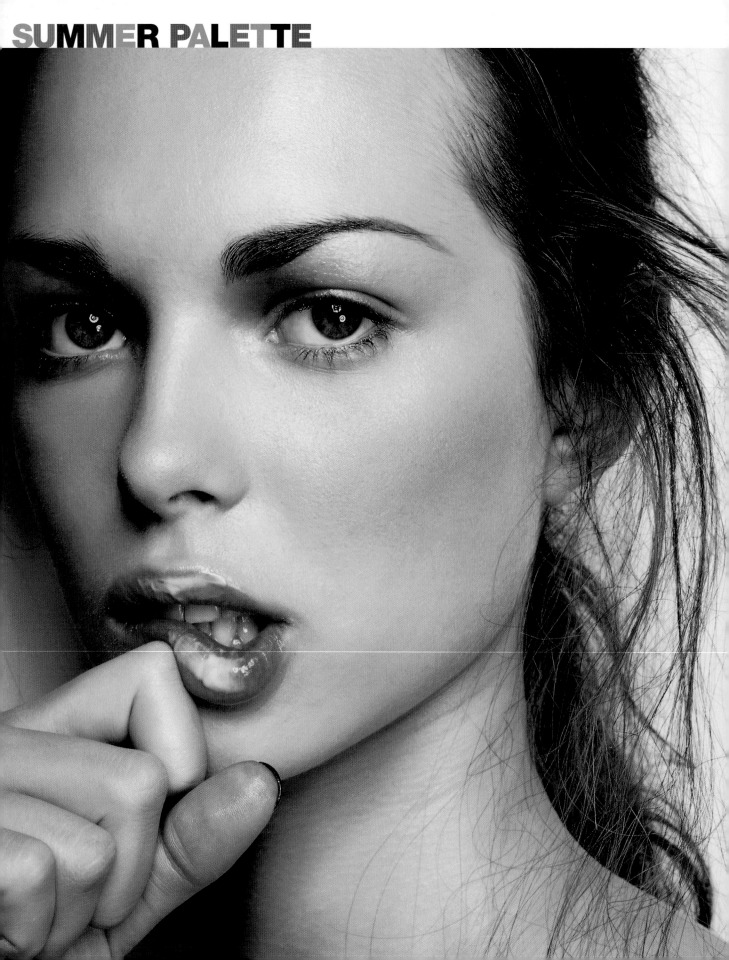

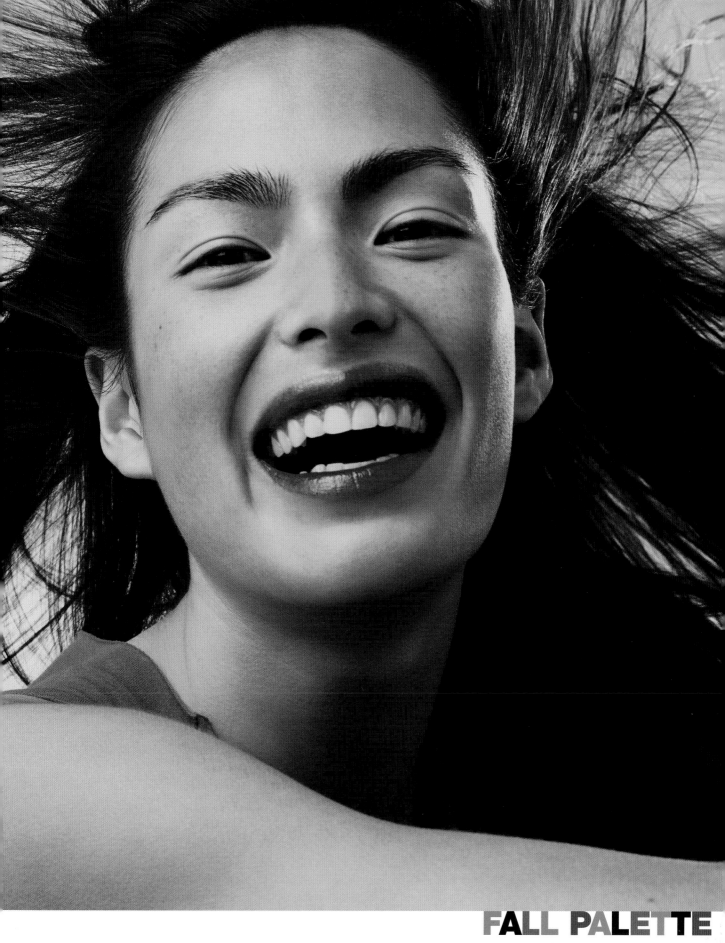

FALL PALETTE

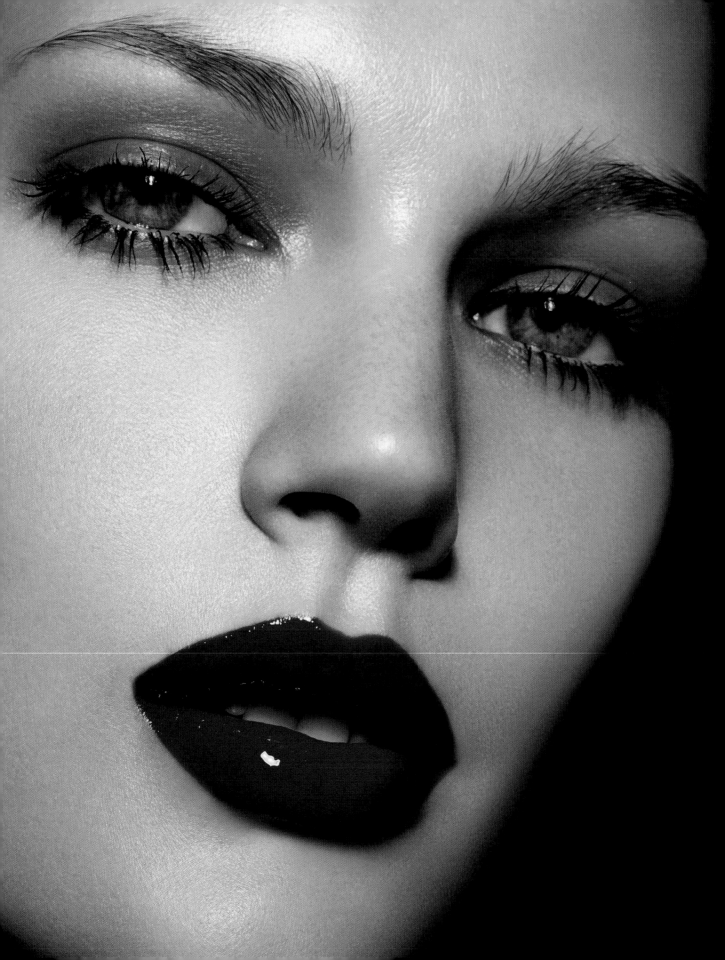

High
beams,
red lights.
Sheer,
full-speed
ahead.

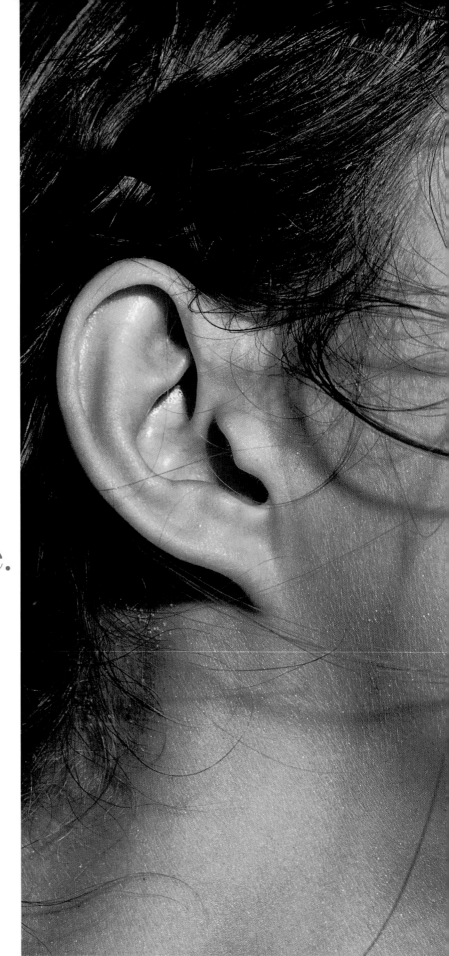

Exquisite.
Sweet
as candy.
Good
enough to
eat.

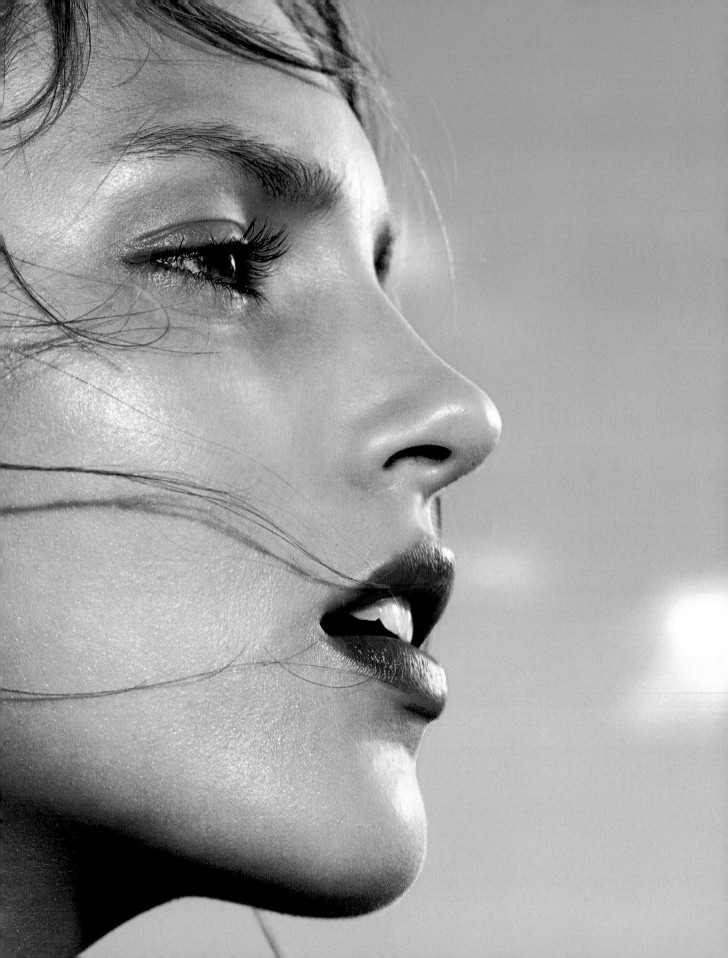

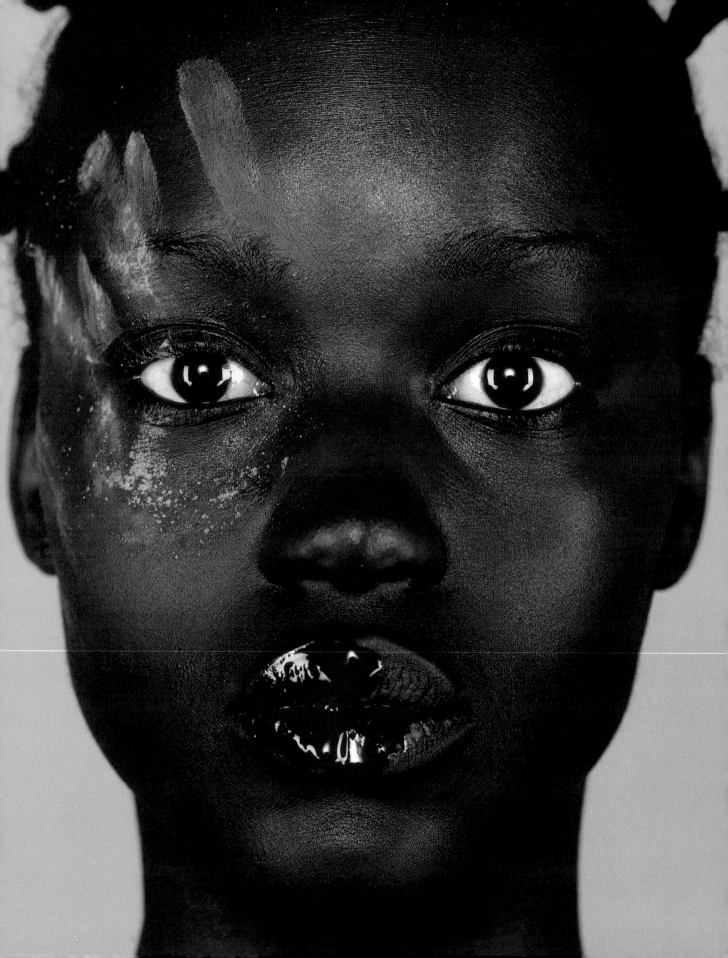

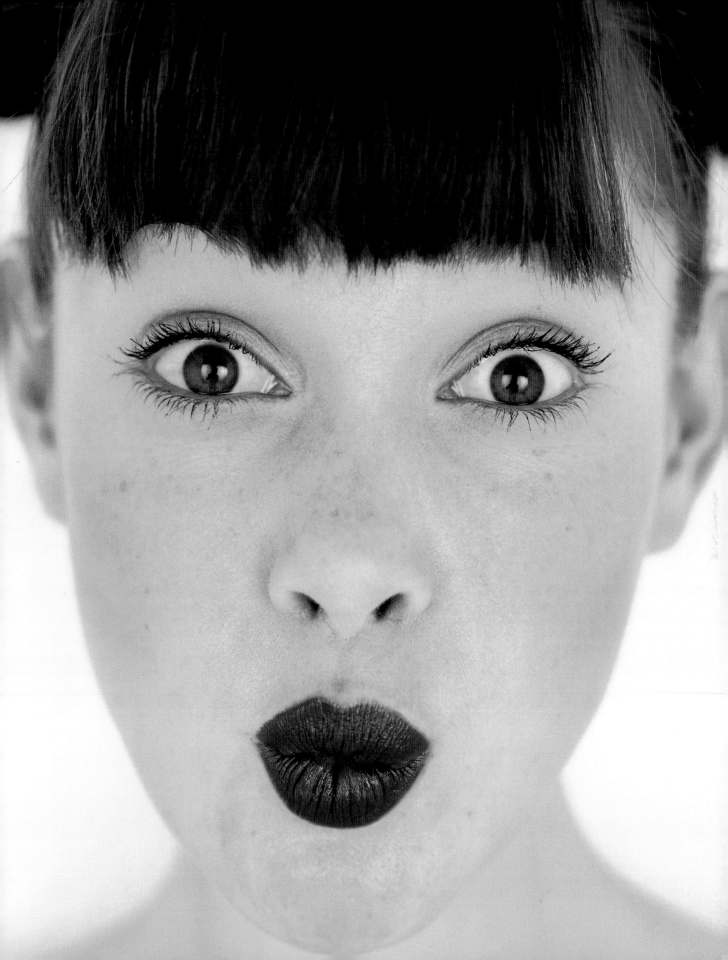

Fire engine red or sensual nude?

What's important in choosing a lipstick? Your complexion, the color of your eyes and hair, the shape of your mouth ... But there are exceptions to every rule. Down with stereotypes and up with making yourself feel good, in every color!

BLONDE OR BRUNETTE Don't believe everything you're told! A bold red can be sublime on a blonde, just like beige can be gorgeous on a brunette.

We aren't living in a monochrome world anymore (matching lips, blush and eye shadow). Instead, you should be shooting for detail. If you're going to accentuate your lips, then compensate by going easy on your eye makeup.

SMALL MOUTHS You're better off with a very light shade like beige (or nude) with which you can cheat on thickness. A color that's too dark tends to accentuate the thinness of your lips.

PLUMP LIPS call for darker shades that will paradoxically draw attention away from your mouth.

Don't be afraid of **bold colors!** It is up to you. **The glossier your lipstick, the easier it will be to wear.** Matte lipsticks can make your face look harsh while ultra-flattering glossy lipsticks bring out the best in your lips. Deep red lipstick is a miracle maker: it will make your teeth appear whiter, has a blushing effect and instantly gives you a sophisticated air.

ADVICE FROM NOLWENN DU LAZ (Journalist at Marie Claire): You want to try a new color for that special evening? Test it during the day and see what reactions you get. If you get the thumbs up, you're ready for a night out on the town!

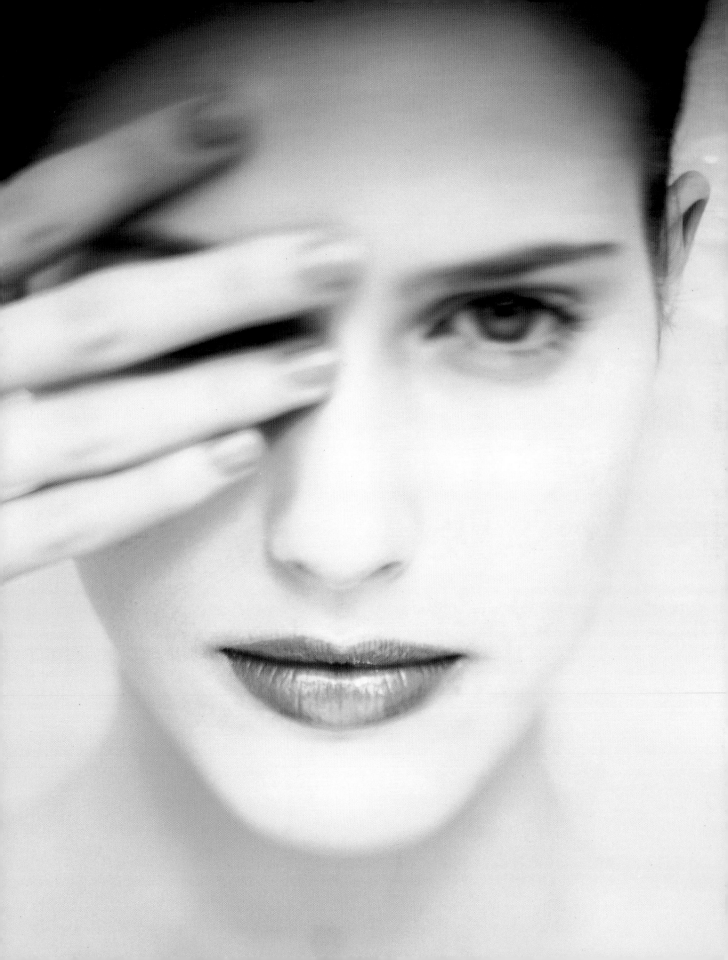

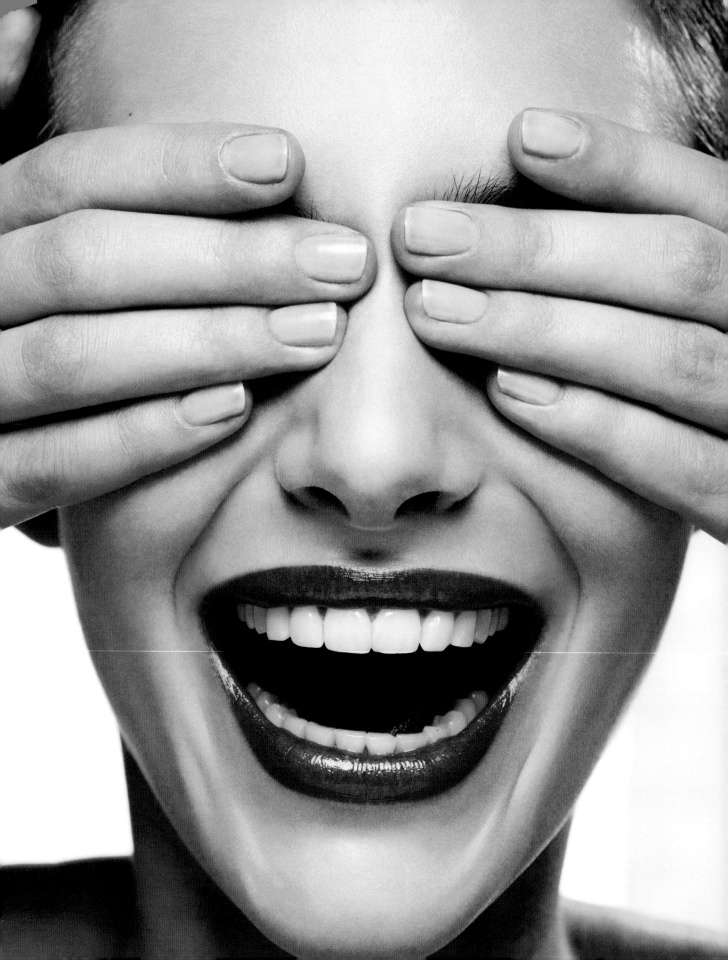

Fingers vs. pencils

How to apply your lipstick is a fundamental question: You need color without thickness! Don't forget your lipliner, a faithful fix-it-all friend who knows how to be subtle.

1 USING YOUR FINGERS For a natural, deliberately imperfect design that is soft and muted, apply lipstick to the flat of your index finger and delicately dab on color from one corner of your mouth to the other — without forgetting the interior of the lip — for an irresistible "just kissed" look.

2 LIP PENCILS are not only for lining the lip: they also help prevent your lipstick from bleeding and from collecting in the small wrinkles around your mouth. Lip pencils will also help you achieve a more matte look. You can even them out with your finger.

TIPS FOR A PERFECT POUT IF YOU HAVE

... droopy lips Try a touch of concealer around both corners of your mouth before lining your lips with a pencil, moving along towards your upper lip

... small lips Try a thin line of beige lip pencil just beyond the natural lines of your mouth, thinning towards the inside of your lips in order to go past your natural lip line with color. Stick with light colors and iridescent formulas

... full lips Try a layer of foundation on the entire mouth, a thin pencil line within the contours of your lips filled in with similar tones with the lightest shade near the corners of your mouth. Avoid dark colors: with full lips, they attract attention but not necessarily in a good way.

ADVICE FROM TERRY (by Terry) — The mille feuille secret: For a spectacular multi-layered effect. After applying your lipstick, use a thick pencil to draw a series of vertical lines across your lips before applying a second coat of lipstick. Top it off with a final swipe of pencil to keep it all in place. You'll achieve excellent hold and the fantastic illusion of fuller lips.

What you'll need
- lipstick
- lip pencil

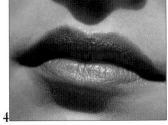
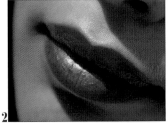
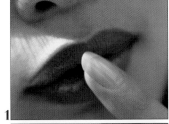
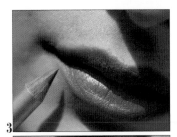
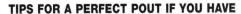

Red: a timeless classic

Immortalized by the noble inspiration of Coco Chanel and reinvented countless times, red lipstick remains the unquestionable mark of ageless elegance.

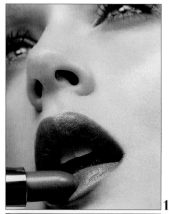

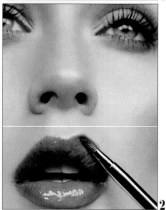

1 VINTAGE REDS ... IN STICKS The flavor of lipstick upon application is the epitome of sensuality and applying it is an act of irresistible femininity. With lipsticks coming in an unending variety of colors and textures, you can put your creativity and imagination to work.

2 DIP YOUR LIP BRUSH Remove lipstick with your finger and "work" it on the back of your hand. This technique has many advantages: warming the product to your body temperature ensures maximal hold. You'll also be able to play with a variety of color nuances in order to achieve a personalized color and extremely flattering three-dimensional effects.

ADVICE FROM A PROFESSIONAL MAKEUP ARTIST (Stilla):
The same lip brush will help you both accent the natural lines of your mouth and color the inside of your lips.

What you'll need
• lipstick
• thin and flat lip brush

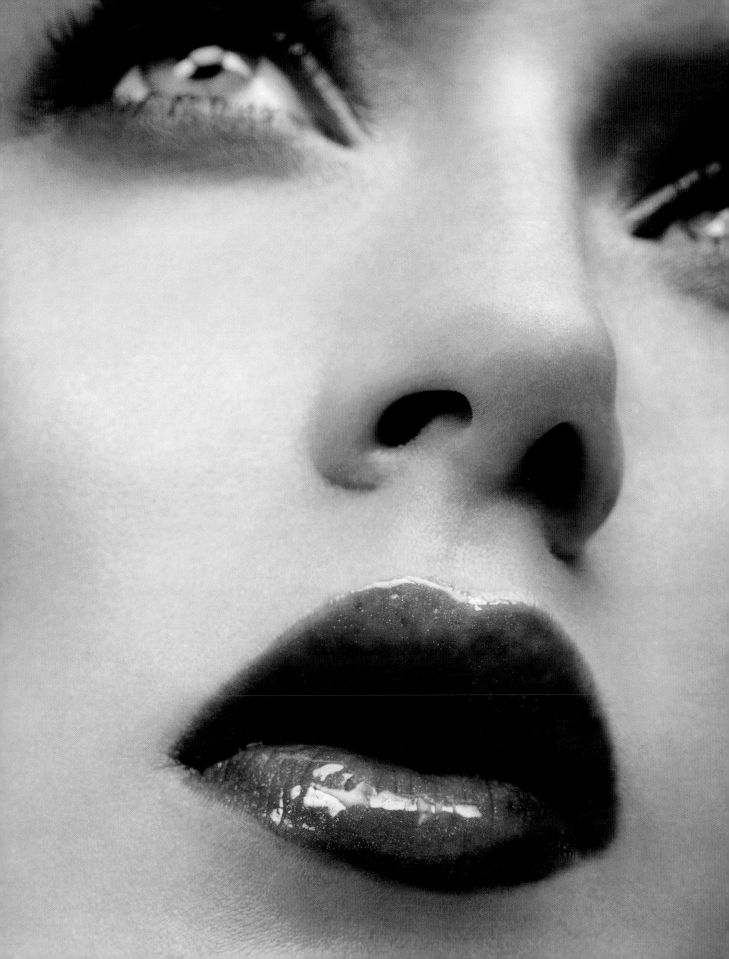

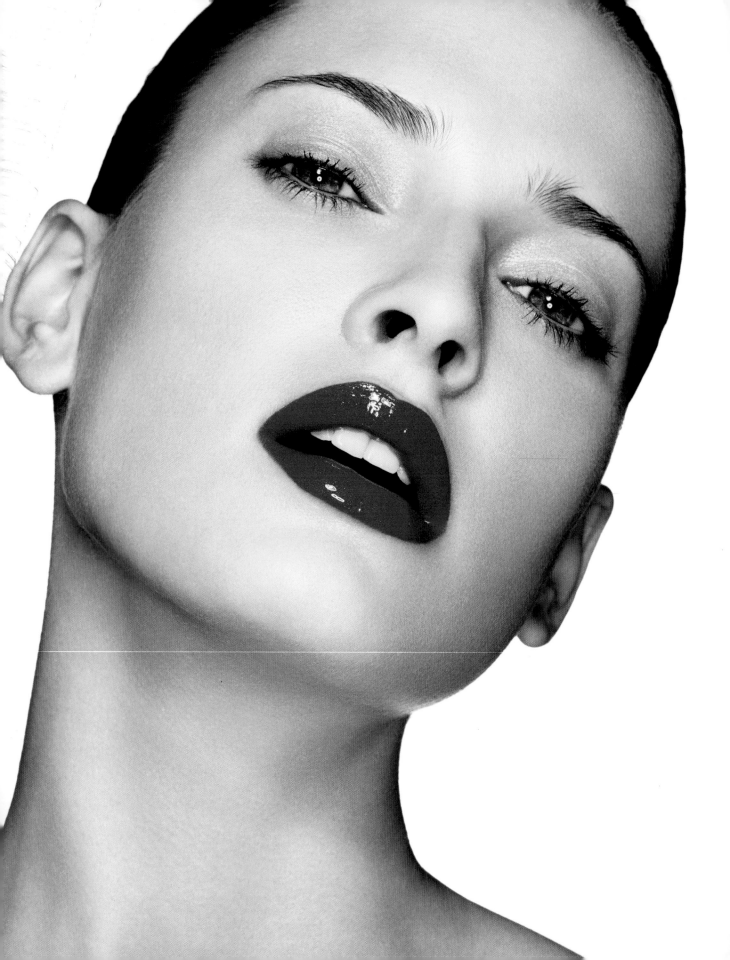

Secrets for luscious lips

Looking for lips as appetizing as juicy fresh fruit? Here are five easy steps to follow for a perfect finish.

1 EXFOLIATE AND EVEN OUT: Like your skin, your mouth also needs to rid itself of dead cells from time to time. Choose a very soft facial exfoliant and gently clean away with a soft, supple toothbrush (reserved exclusively for this purpose) for silky lips.

2 NOURISH: Generously apply an ultra-rich, creamy lip balm (or even Vaseline) for several minutes, then wipe away with a cotton swab.

3 CONTOURS: Think of your lip liner as your lips' guardrails. It should be the same color as your lipstick, but one shade lighter. Nude tones will suit paler complexions and will yield a flattering effect of increased volume.

4 LUSH BRUSH: Coat both sides of the brush with lipstick and start applying from the inside of your lips, moving upwards in small strokes until you reach the outer edges.

5 LET IT SHINE! Lip gloss will help bring it all together: a single dollop in the middle of your lips will create a dynamic three-dimensional effect. Of course you can also spread it across your whole lip for a full-on shine.

What you'll need
- soft-tipped lip pencil
- flat lip brush
- vibrant lipstick
- lip gloss, either clear or the same color as the lipstick

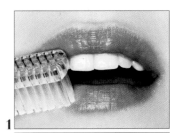

2

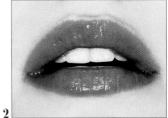

3

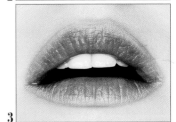

1

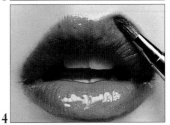

4

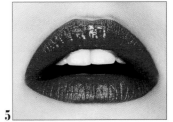

5

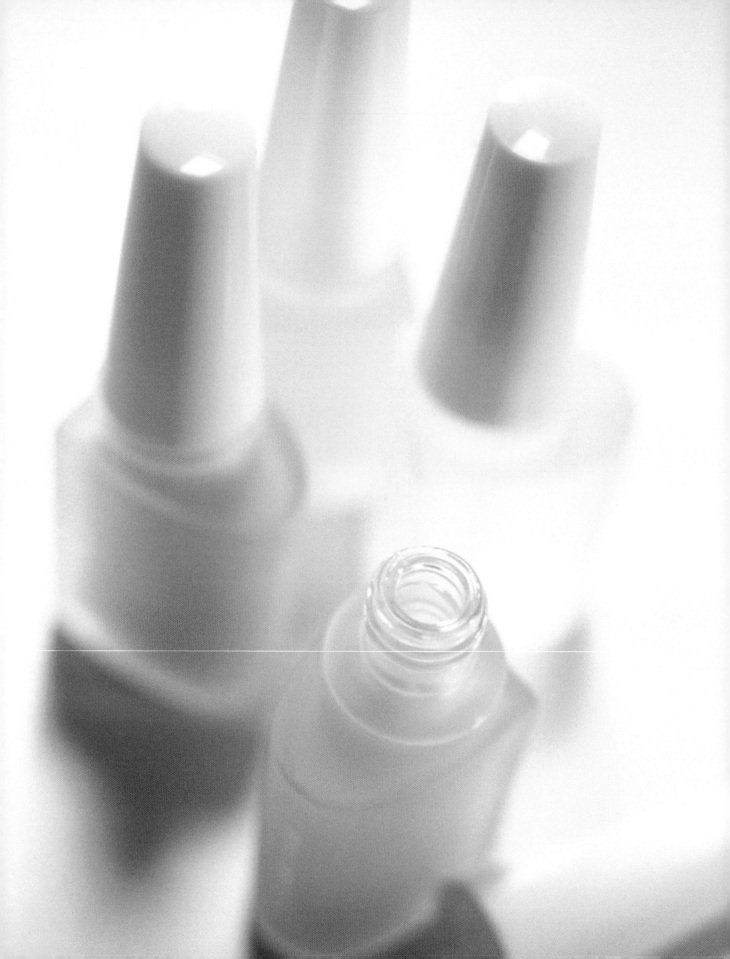

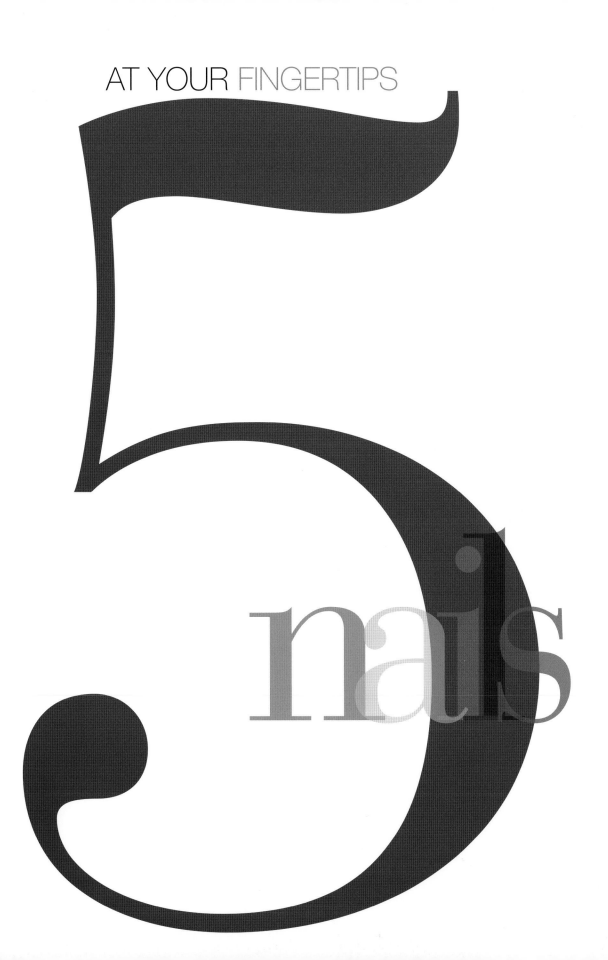

nails

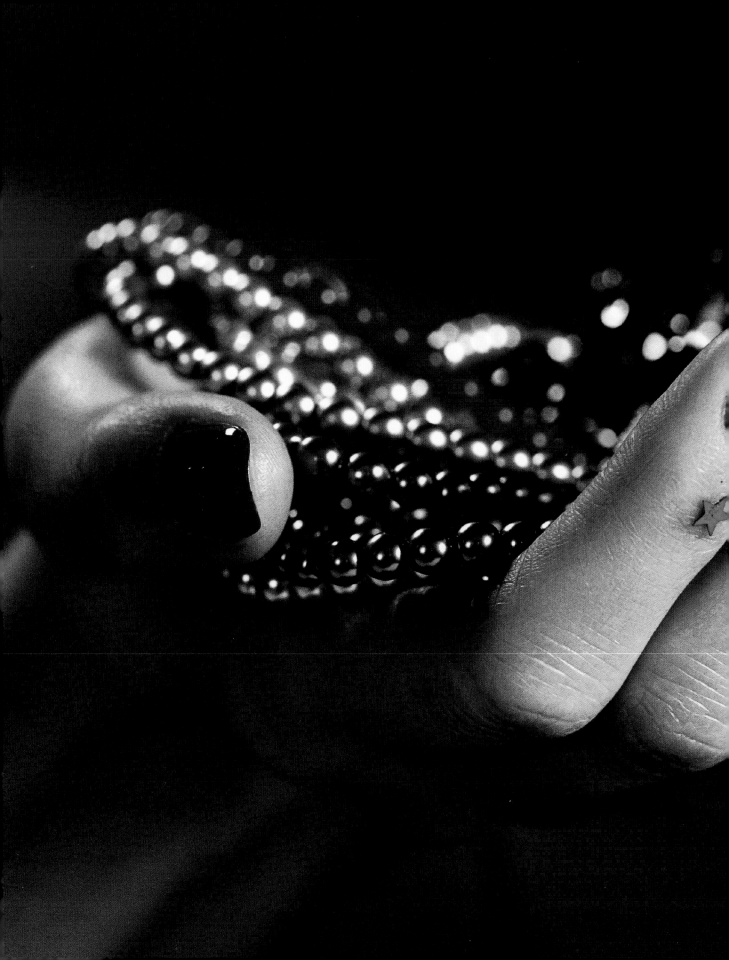

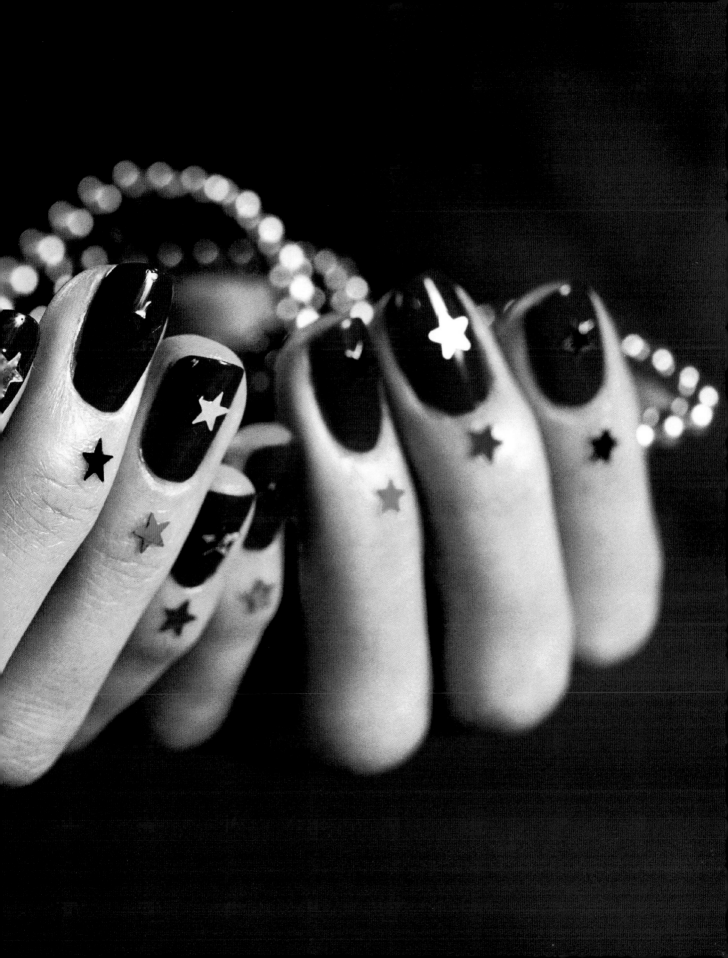

Poppies, pinks and pastels. Perfect pretty palette

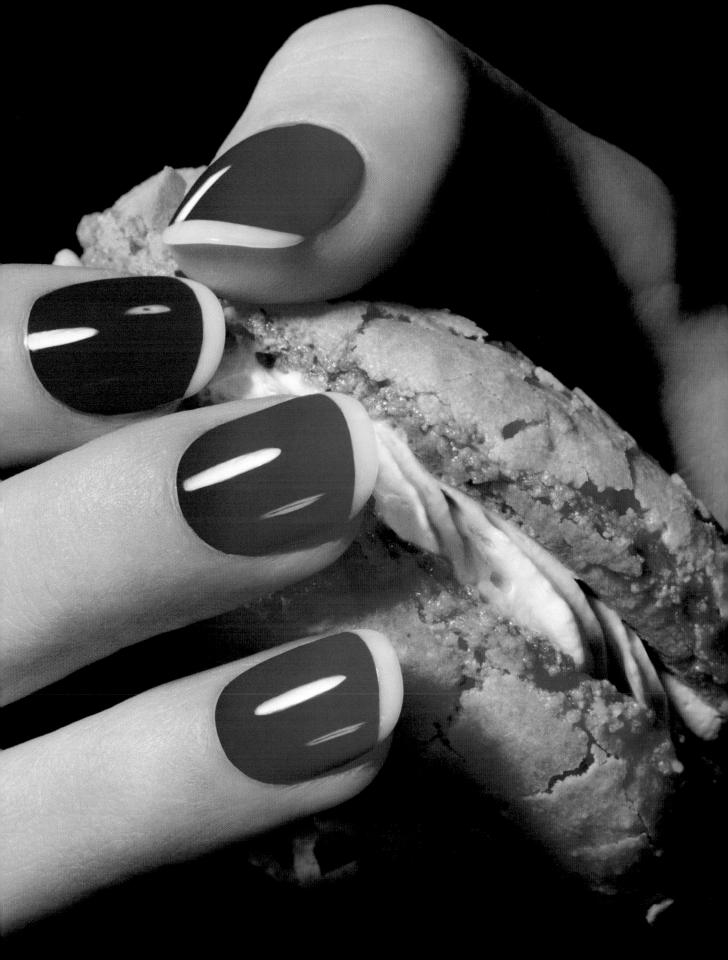

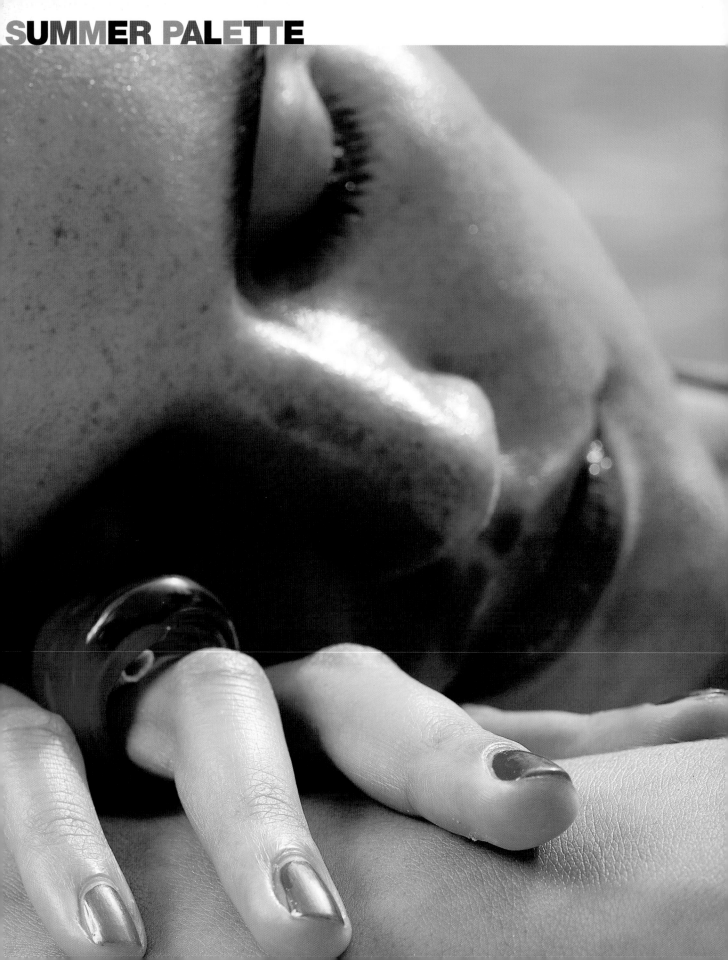

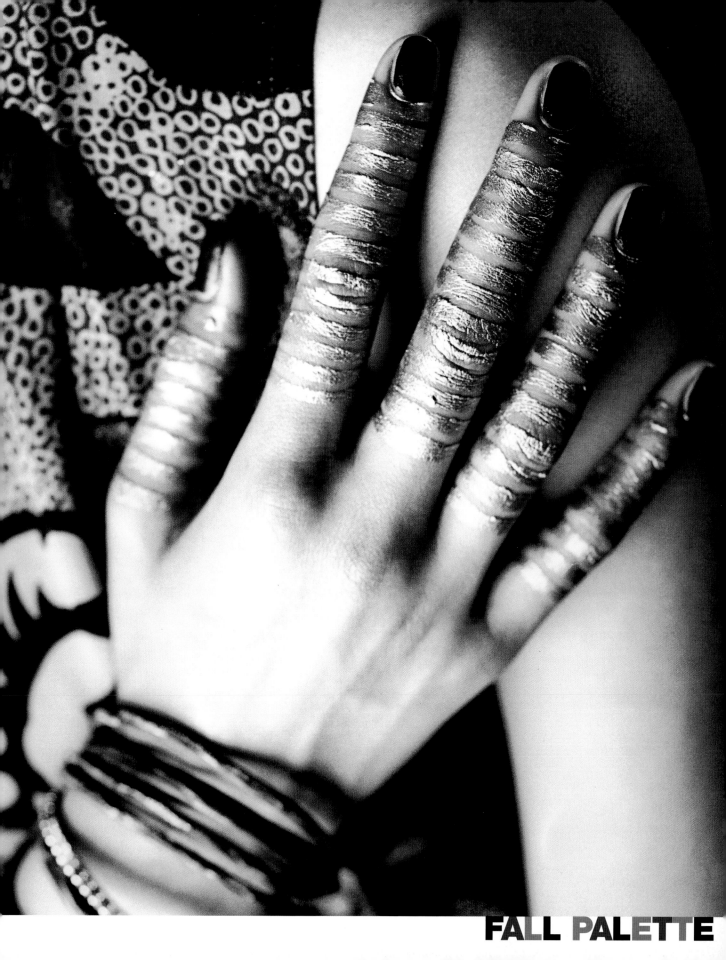

FALL PALETTE

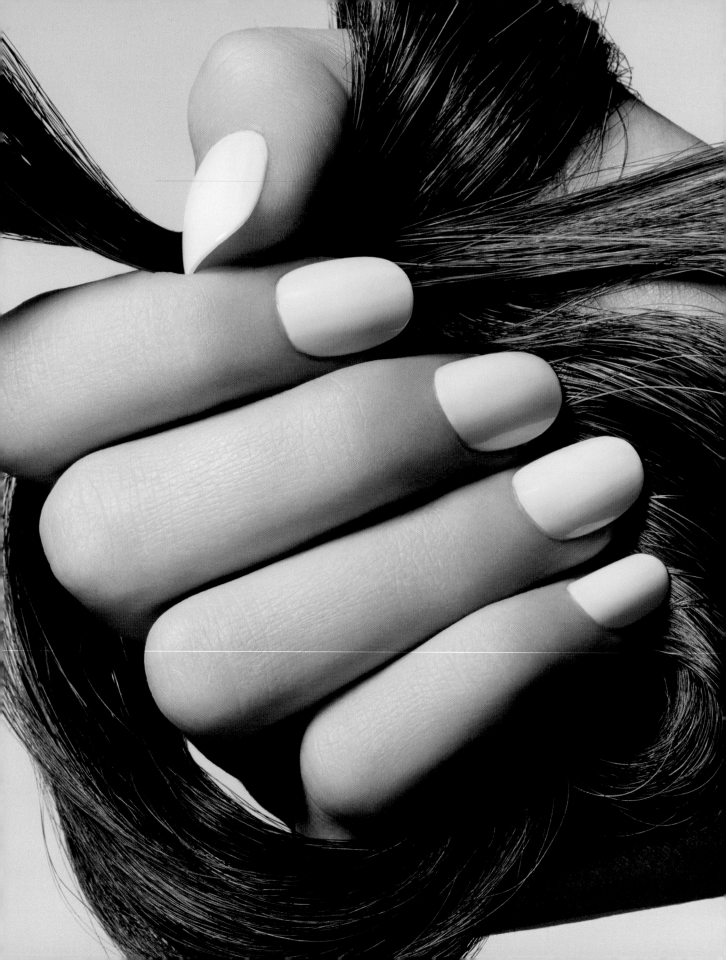

Chic city girls claw their way through town with style and flair.

Express manicure

Nails are anything but simple accessories: chic or shock, they arm your hands with an undeniable power of seduction.

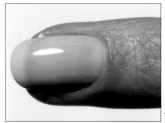

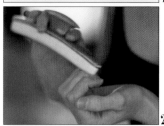

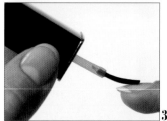

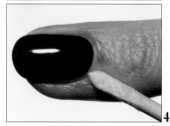

1 PAMPERED HANDS The key to beautiful nails lies in constant care: under the nails should be spotless and your half-moons well cared-for; cuticles should be pushed back and the smallest imperfection taken care of immediately. Daily use of the right nourishing and hydrating cream according to your skin type and age will help. The perfect length? Not too long nor too short, use the shape of your fingertip as a guide. A rounded square shape is always a must.

2 FILING AND BUFFING Your nails should be as buffed as well as a small seashell. Whether or not you're going to use polish, the slightest bump will stick out like a sore thumb!

3 KEEP YOUR BASES COVERED A good base and primer will strengthen and protect your nails.

4 SEXY POLISH With today's products offering ultra-shiny and incredibly vibrant colors at record-breaking drying speed, beautiful nails have never been easier. Let yourself loose! However, beware of flaking and peeling: nothing looks more neglected than chipped nail polish.

ADVICE FROM A PROFESSIONAL NAIL CARE SPECIALIST Gisèle Pommier (L'onglerie):
With one sweep, take just enough polish for one nail and wipe any excess away into the bottle. Contrary to what most people believe, you should start in the middle of your nail, at the edge, fanning downwards to the base, finishing at the sides, leaving a small space on either side.

What you'll need
- orangewood cuticle sticks
- nail file (emery board, glass or ceramic)
- pumice stone
- manicure scissors
- nail clippers
- buffer
- exfoliating cream
- nourishing cream
- nail polish remover
- base and primer, nail polish, top coat and activating spray

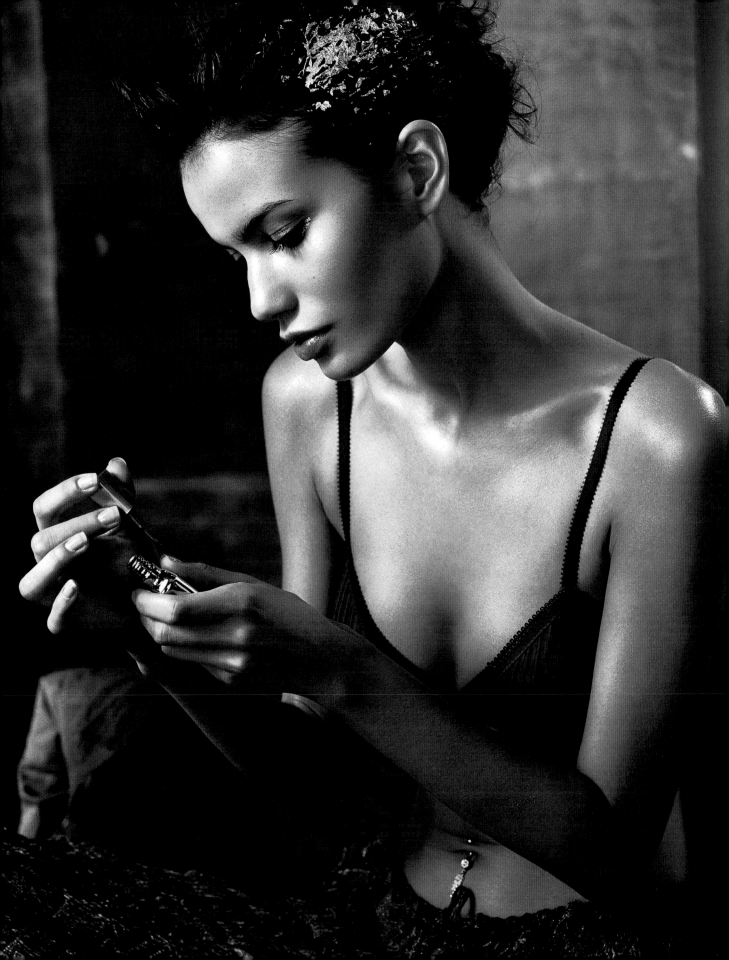

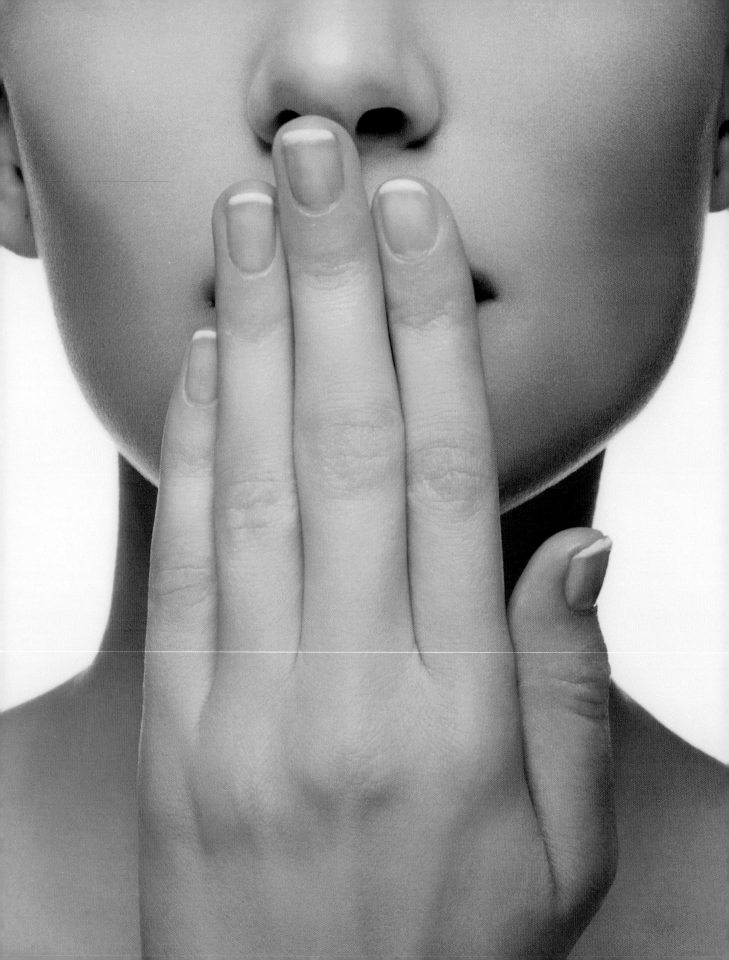

The French manicure: a worldwide winner

Refined and especially flattering against sun-kissed skin, the discreet elegance of the most famous of manicures requires care and attention to detail. Here are some tips to get you on the right track.

1 FILE THE NAIL rather short, once completely cleaned of old polish, either in a slightly squared or round shape.

2 REMOVE HANGNAILS with manicure scissors. After applying a cuticle softening cream, push your cuticles back with a wood cuticle stick.

3 Delicately **APPLY WHITE POLISH** to nail tips, following the natural tip of the nails. You can try adhesive guide strips or a kit with a curved brush: any excess polish can be removed with a nail polish remover stick.

4 APPLY BEIGE OR PINK POLISH as soon as the opaque polish on the tips has completely dried. Cover your entire nail with clear polish which will give the white tips a more natural look. Once you've got the hang of it, you can try to give yourself a colored French manicure (see page 130) or replace the white tips with gold or silver, for a party, for example.

5 A TOP COAT that protects while it shines is the essential last touch for an irresistibly impeccable finish. It will also help increase the durability of your manicure. Top it off with a nourishing cream or oil.

ADVICE FROM ODILE SIBUET (manicurist): French manicure kits are extremely practical: covering the nail plate, they leave just the tips exposed, helping you to paint a perfect half-moon. Wait until the white polish is completely dry before removing the tip guide.

What you'll need
- nail file
- orangewood cuticle sticks
- cuticle cream
- white opaque polish
- beige or pink nail polish
- top coat

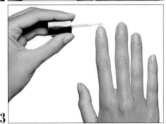

1

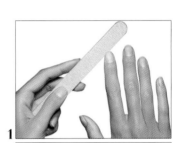

2

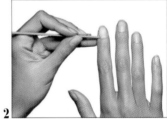

3

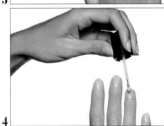

4

5

Your best foot forward

As soon as the sun comes out, you break out your sandals and show the world your feet. Here are a few tips for beautiful feet from an expert podiatrist and pedicurist.

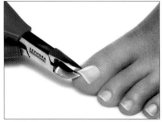

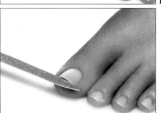

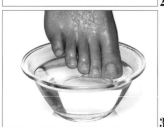

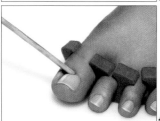

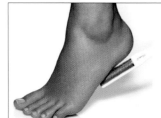

1 **CUT** your toenails with clippers and even them out into a rounded square shape with a nail file. Beware of cutting the corners too short as this can lead to ingrown nails.

2 **EXFOLIATE THEN SOAK** your feet for 10 minutes in a warm bath of aromatherapy oils, bath balls or epsom salts. Use this time to scrub your toenails.

3 As soon as you remove your foot from the bath, or after dipping your toes in emollient, **PUSH BACK** your cuticles with an orangewood cuticle stick. Next, buff your nails with an abrasive buffer and then apply nail oil to the whole nail, paying particular attention to the nail bed.

4 Use a foot file or a wet pumice stone to **SLOUGH AWAY** calluses and dead skin cells on the balls and heels of your feet. Some corns can be removed with keratolytic cream (use very carefully). If in doubt, quickly make an appointment with your podiatrist!

5 Give your feet a long massage using your favorite moisturizer (hydrating or cooling). Using a cotton swab dipped in nail polish remover, get rid of any greasy residue on your toes. You're now ready to attempt a French pedicure (see page 137)!

ADVICE FROM ARI DARMON (Podiatrist and pedicurist):
Using a home foot spa with rollers will add to the relaxing aspect of your pedicure. Even without polish, your toenails can shine with a "supershine" buffer. Wrapping a bit of cotton on the end of your cuticle sticks will make pushing skin back less painful and, if dipped in nail polish remover, will also help you clean up after any application errors. To separate your toes, use a rolled-up facial tissue: it's practical and hygienic. Be sure to always dry between your toes to avoid cracks and fungal infections. Finally, be sure to put on your pedicure slippers before you start painting your toenails!

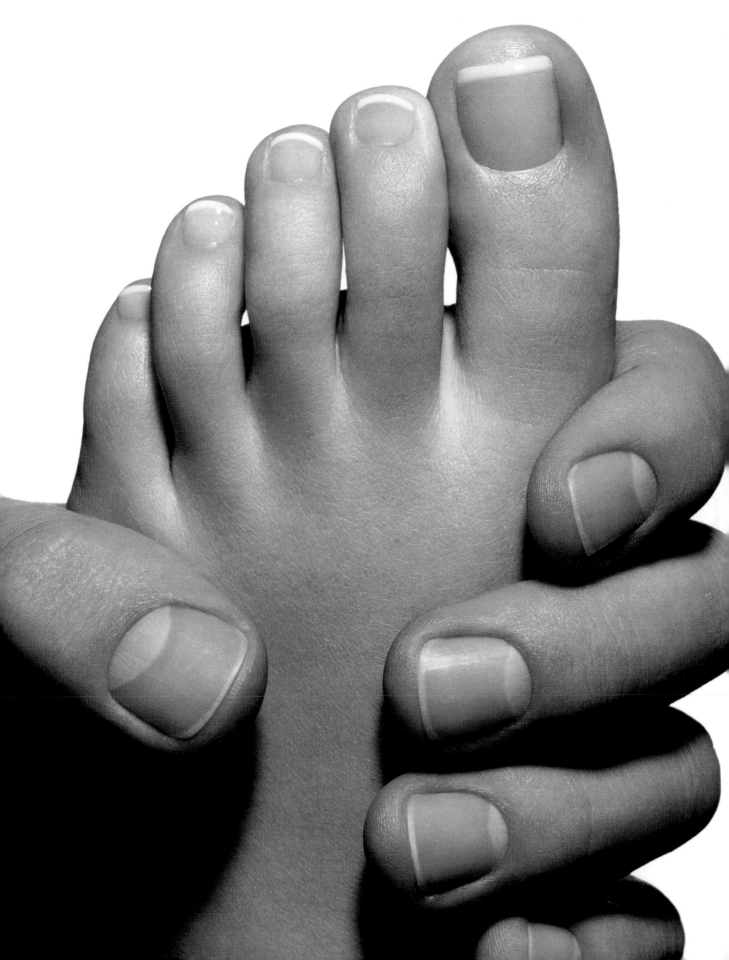

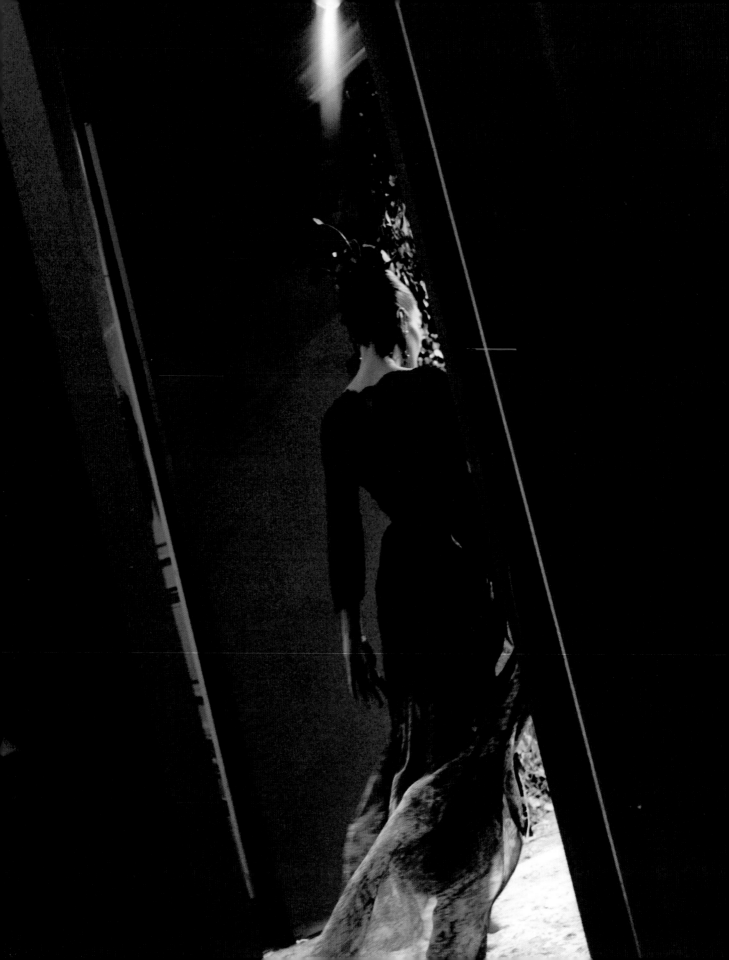

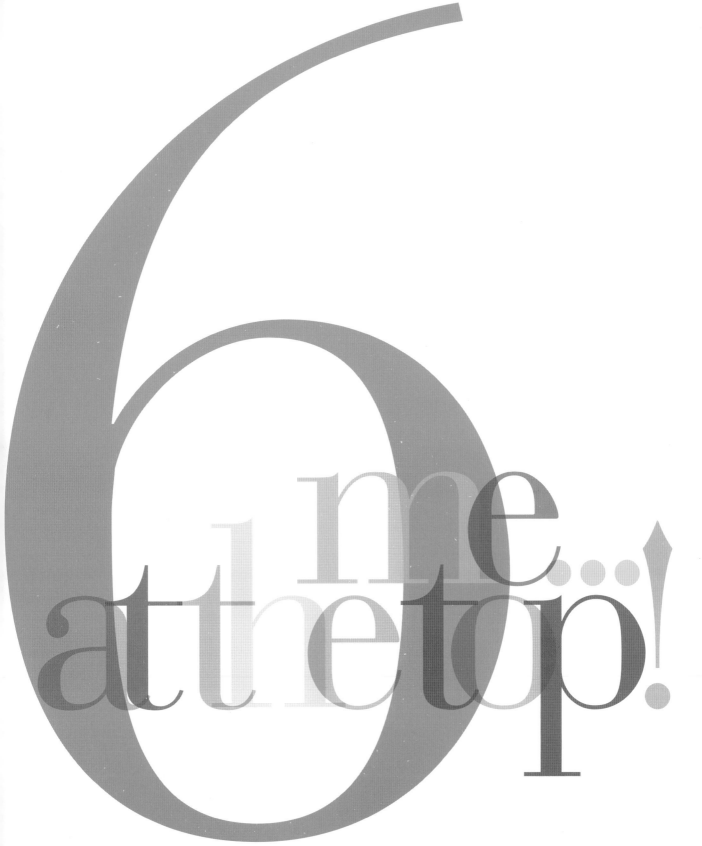

6 me at the top...!

MAKEUP ARTISTS' TRADE SECRETS

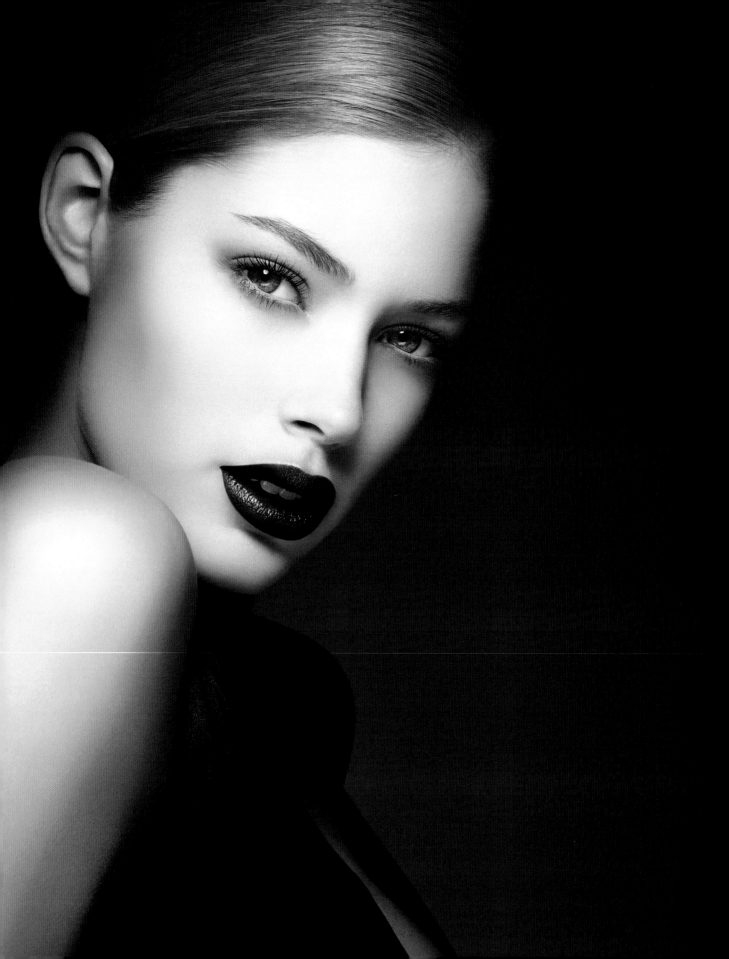

Olivier Echaudemaison
Creative Director, Guerlain

A makeup artist whose address book would make any celebrity-watcher's face pale, Olivier Echaudemaison is adored by queens, princesses and celebrities the world over. Nonetheless, he has maintained a crucial distance and sense of humor that are the key to his absolute elegance. His take on beauty is a lesson in humanity …

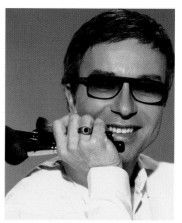

"The one thing to bring to a desert island? Lipstick!"

Beauty is a timeless concept; it has nothing to do with short-lived trends or fads. That is why I prefer to talk about style rather than fashion. So why change when you've found yours? Trying to look like someone else is proof of insecurity … But today, we don't know how to look at ourselves anymore, we see ourselves only in pieces. It's time to rediscover an overall vision of ourselves. This is why I love 'before and after' makeovers —the only problem is when the 'before' is better than the 'after'!

In my forty years in the makeup industry, in spite of all the new gadgets, nothing has really changed: we still have eyes and lips. **How you wear your eyeliner or your lipstick is reassuring and self-affirming. After all, you're naked without it!**

Cosmetic products are only as interesting as the stories they tell: how do they seduce and attract all the senses? How aesthetically pleasing are they? How sensuous to the touch? Even the sounds of the clasps and the perfumes count: you can recognize the unmistakable violet scent of Guerlain with your eyes closed, for example.

Without spending too much, you can indulge in boundless luxury, self-gratification and a certain social status associated with a strong image.

On the other hand, what has changed are the formulas and the ways we apply makeup: the invention of weightlessness and radiance. Guerlain has illustrated this tendency with the creation of Meteorites and especially Terracotta, a twenty year-old revolution: makeup that you can't see.

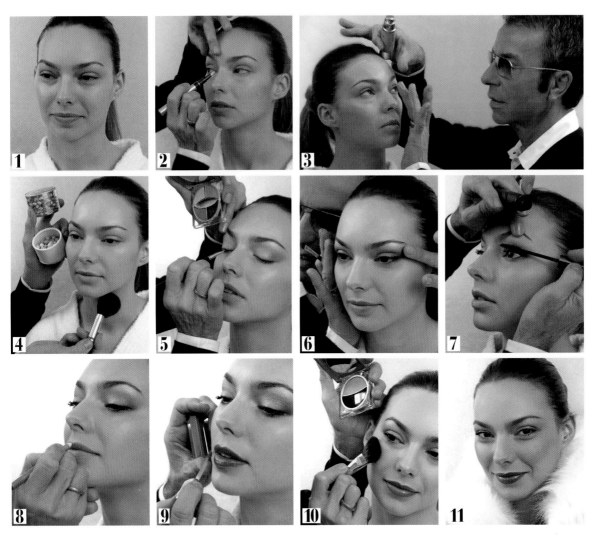

MID-SEASON MAKEUP. 1. Use an intense hydrating cream on your clean face. 2. Moisturizing foundation with Active Rose Extract for a natural and flawless complexion. 3. Apply stick concealer in the inner corner under your eye. For more effective blending with with your skin, smoothen with your fingertips from the inner corner to the outer one. 4. For a superb complexion, use Meteorites Powder for the Face. Gold and mother-of-pearl brings harmonious radiance and translucency. Brighten your complexion by dipping the brush in the beads and applying over the whole face, neck and shoulders, paying particular attention to the nose, chin and forehead. 5. Eye makeup with Ombre Eclat Eyeshadow, four delicate beige shades that create a mysterious look. The "Lighter" shadow makes the eyes dazzle with a pearly sparkle. "Velvet" complements beige taupe. With the "Medium" you can create depth with misty grays by applying it to the crease of your eyelid and up to the brow bone. Finally, use "Contour" and its sparkly black to add structure, definition and radiance. 6. Larger eyes. 7. Final (and indispensable) step: mascara. Maxi Lash — Extreme Volume Mascara will give depth and volume to your lashes. 8. Guerlain's secret for sensual lips is the Divinora Ivoire Cupid Lip Pencil. To highlight the cupid's arrow of your upper lip a touch of light in the middle, like a kiss curl. 9. For a shiny, lacquered effect, use KissKiss Laquer — Intense Glossy Finish Fabulous Rose. Smooth and thick, this gloss goes on easily thanks to its sponge brush. 10. Blush is the final touch, after applying your lipstick. This helps you judge the color's intensity: this is Divinora Radiant Blush in Rose Pluie d'Or, fresh as a rose petal.
11. The result: makeup that is both soft and sophisticated.

"When looking at Ava Gardner onscreen, women could snatch a beauty recipe or two!"

When a woman says, "I don't use makeup, I just use Terracotta," it makes me laugh! This spectacular technological revolution is to makeup what microfibers and spandex were to fashion. Movement is no longer the same.

What this means for you is that you don't have to be an expert anymore to do your own makeup. Years ago, cosmetics were hard to manipulate and women made mistakes. It was a difficult art, reserved for a precious few, such as actresses and socialites. Besides these and other worldly women, who got made up professionally, rare were those women who could afford such luxury.

Nevertheless, since time immemorial, Parisian women have found solutions. French women are good cooks and as far as beauty is concerned, they know that all you need is a good recipe!

Think of it as the communal beauty kitchen: while admiring such great performers as Ava Gardner or Sylvie Vartan, French women were able to steal a trick or two for themselves.

Elsewhere in the world, approaches to female beauty are much more stereotyped than in France. They are also very telling about culture: just look at Asian pinks, rice powder and whitening techniques (the cultural acceptance of sun tanning was revolutionary at the time).

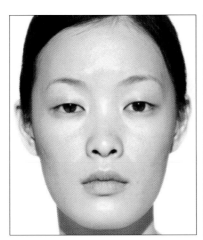 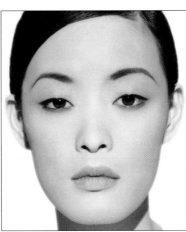 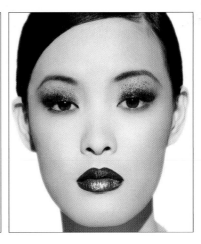

HEIN, STYLED BY OLIVIER ECHAUDEMAISON in three spectacular steps: 1. Before. 2. For daytime: a foundation that creates a seamless complexion, eyebrows redrawn with a pencil, eyes highlighted with beige eyeshadow and lifted by a touch of black eyeliner, shiny rose lipstick. 3. For evening: glitter and more daring colors for shadow that is overlaid and blended, a touch of lipliner, lipstick, and a dash of blush give the final accents.

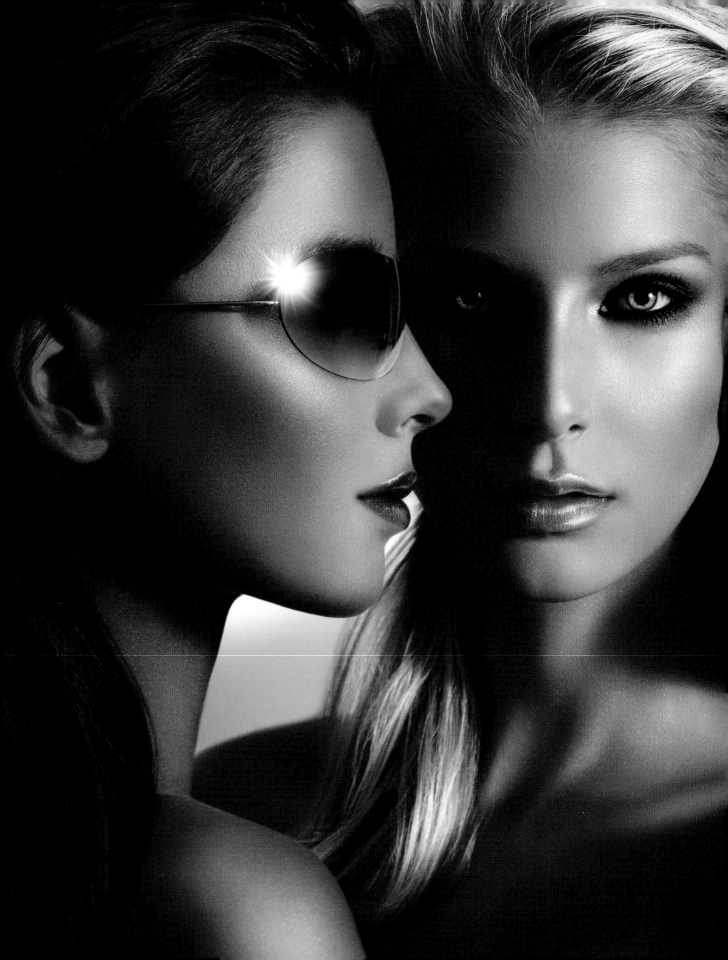

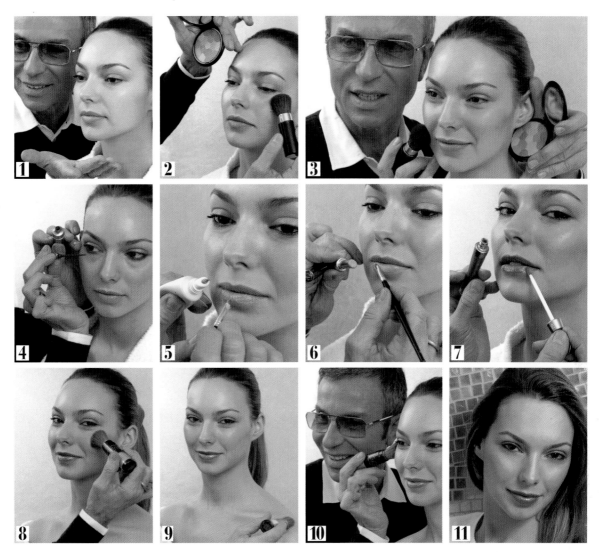

SUN-KISSED BEAUTY LESSON. 1. Fully hydrate your skin with Super Aqua-Day Refreshing Gel-Cream. 2. Highlight certain features such as your cheekbones or your eyebrow arch by applying Terracotta Light Sheer Bronzing Powder with a brush. It comes in two palettes named "Blondes" for pale blondes (soft and elegant glow) and "Brunettes" for olive-skinned women (who will look like they've just returned from the Caribbean). 3. A bright and natural complexion thanks to a harmonious blend of five shades that guarantees a radiant mien. 4. For a captivating, sensual and downright fascinating look, use Terracotta Loose Powder Kohl. Like all kohls, it can be applied on the eyelid as well as on the inner lower lid. An easy color to wear, it opens up the expressions of blondes and brunettes alike without hardening your face; it simply leaves you mysteriously sexy. 5. For perfectly moisturized lips, use a brush to apply Divinora Lipbalm before lipstick or gloss. 6. To prep your lips for lipstick and ensure long-lasting color, use Liplift Beautifying Fixative. 7. For a soft and radiant smile, choose a shade from Gloss & Shine. 8. An amber shade blush to make your tan effervescent. 9. To have a sensual glow, caress your face and body with Meteorites Pearly Touch Powder (limited edition that comes in two shades, Blondes #1 with highlights or Brunettes #2 with copper highlights). 10. To get people to pay attention to you, apply to strategic zones such as your neck, shoulders, arms and ankles. 11. A bright sun-kissed look that lasts for hours. **Result, on the opposite page: a sun-kissed face and body, a signature look of the timeless Terracotta line,** composed of brown, copper and golden nuances.

"Foundation is as intimate as lingerie — as close to your skin as it gets."

While French mothers tend to forbid makeup at a young age, American mothers work better in guilt, pushing their daughters to mask imperfections ("Hide your pimples and you'll have a date for the prom!"). On the other hand, "neutral" is the name of the game: from foundation to lipstick, everything is beige in America these days.

Today's makeup is elusive — secret and imperceptible. If you can see the work that goes into it, then you haven't succeeded …

Foundation is as intimate as lingerie — as close to your skin as it gets. If it's poorly chosen it can become the ugliest thing in the world: it could harden like a mask and make you look grainy. What's more (and this is what makes product development so fascinating these days) is that it can be practically invisible today. **People shouldn't say to you, "What a lovely foundation you're wearing today!" but rather "Your skin looks beautiful today!"**

As for your lips, they can live their own life — red, purple or gothic black — because they show the color of your mood. They also affirm your sensuality, not to mention your sexuality: men won't ever put makeup on their lips!

Lips have always been a fashion accessory: during the miniskirt crazy of the 1960s, leggings were yoghurt-colored and lips were pearly-whitened to makeup for the sexed-up leg exposure. It was a way of toning down any sexual connotation of the lips. In the 1970s, when mid-length and long skirts came back in style, lips were done in copper and brown!

A pant-wearing woman without makeup is a man. But the same woman, in the same outfit with heels and red lips is a knockout!

The one thing to bring to a desert island? Lipstick! And that's it!

The French name for lipstick, "rouge à lèvres," is too restrictive — why limit the name of this fabulous product to just one color? Let's keep to more English names, like gloss, or even lip makeup.

A cultish object, lipstick is an incredible weapon of seduction. If a woman chooses to use it in public, and if the act of using it is beautiful to behold, the object itself must be as well. KissKiss, Guerlain's signature lipstick that I put back out on the market with Van Straten's help, is timeless and sensual. It's unbelievable to think that it has conquered 17 per cent of the worldwide market!

Women are attracted to its name, its color, and its shape. We're not talking about consumerism … we're talking about instinct and pure pleasure.

A snow princess straight out of a fairytale showcases a winter palette.

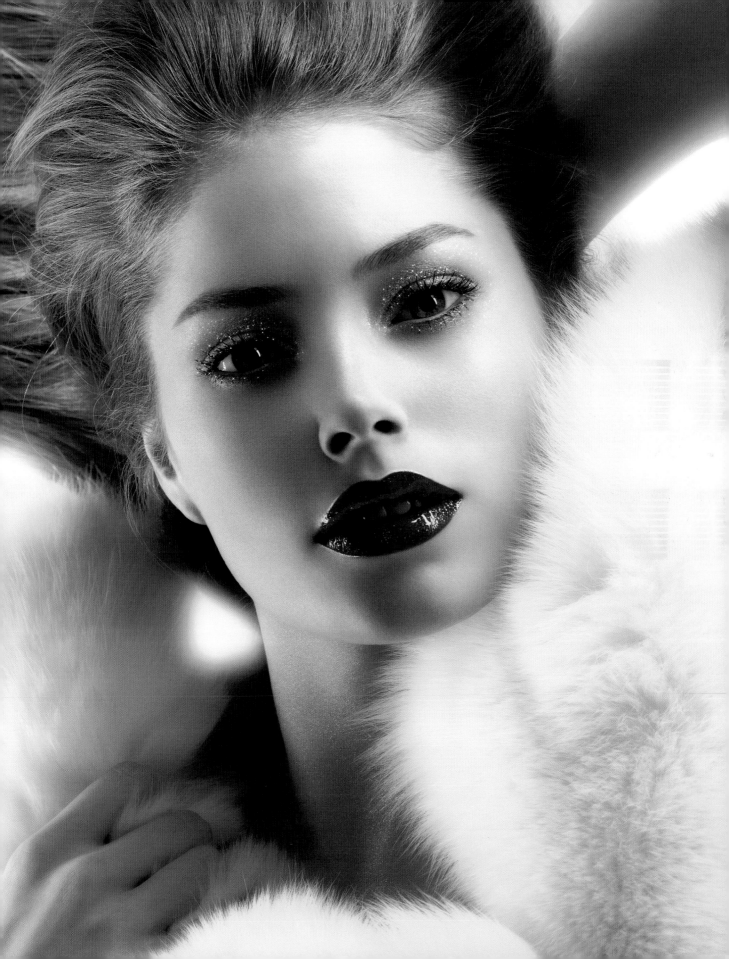

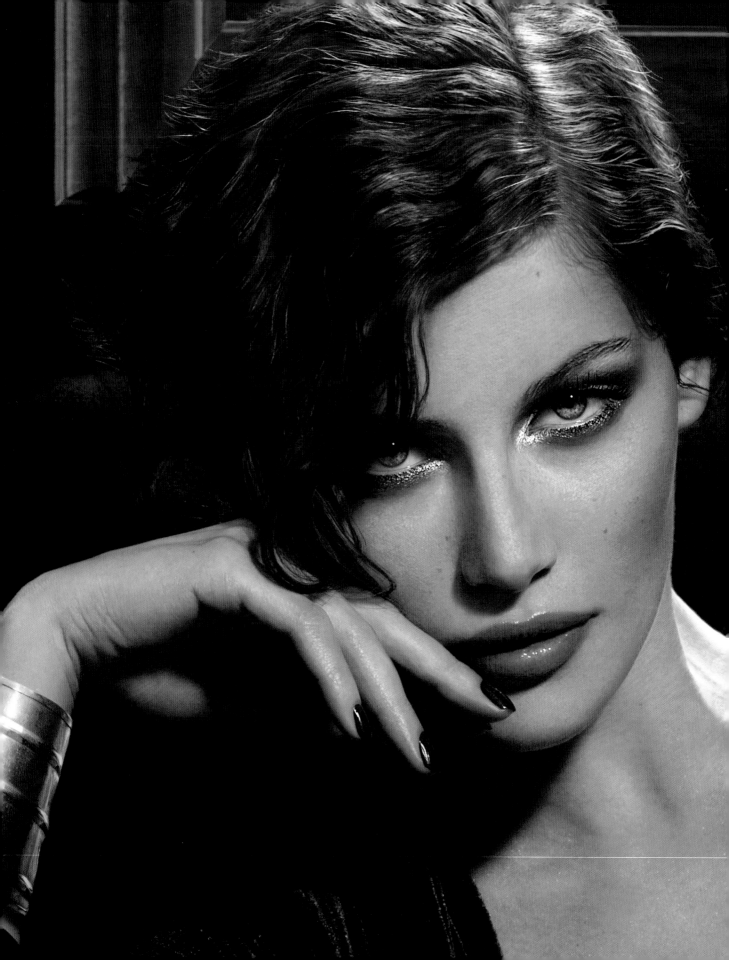

James Kaliardos
Makeup Artist at L'Oréal Paris

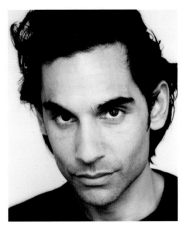

James Kaliardos is an artist of feeling: he holds the faces of the women he makes up in high esteem and is interested in the person as a whole. Unknown or world-renowned, he conquers every woman he works on thanks to his translucent art that falls somewhere between spectacular and natural. Each perfect detail contributes to one singular image — and it is always sublime.

"Makeup is a strong **medium** for effectively **revealing** something **unique** about **yourself** that comes from within …"

Nothing forces a woman to make herself up or have her hair done — these are only means to an end; strong ways to effectively reveal something unique about yourself that comes from within … and these acts also help give you the confidence to make a statement.

Clearly there has been a revolution around how women relate to beauty — I have been working on a project where I study the role of beauty in women's lives by decade. I did not go into this totally unknowledgeable, I already knew what these changes meant but did not understand the fundamental reasons behind them. Generally speaking, throughout history, as wars have broken out, women have been pushed 'behind the scenes'. At war's end, they come back out to the forefront, feeling the need to have a pronounced look that is often rather 'extreme'.

We're lucky today to be living in a time of freedom where women can actually choose how they want to look. Makeup can be 'trendy', not wearing it can be, too. Wearing your hair straight is in vogue as much a tousled, straight-out-of-bed look.

But **women living in the 1950s were forced to wear thick foundation, red lipstick and eyeliner** and to get perms at the hairdresser's — in a word, an odd style by today's standards. There were some frankly unattractive women back then, and you practically couldn't look at them. That type of look is not for everyone!"

Laetitia Casta, the ultimate muse, is the epitome of ideal beauty and a true, albeit revisited nature.

"Your 'look' only counts for 20 per cent. What's essential is your personality, your way of being ..."

Now imagine yourself in the sixties: you would need an extra half-hour per day to put on your false eyelashes. Men have never had these types of constraints.

All that is over now — today, you can do as you please! This represents true power for today's women — a crucial victory, even though we must not forget that in some places of the world, women are not allowed to show their faces.

Sometimes I work on photo shoots where the models are treated horribly, posing in a dark alley or on a staircase like some poor streetwalker. I am ferociously against that. Is it really necessary to paint beautiful women in this light? It is all the more shocking when you consider that these women are often the ones who run the magazines their pictures appear in. I fight constantly against these types of images and believe in more noble representations of women. **A woman can be truly strong and beautiful at the same time. I think that beauty is a power that men will never have.** Women have their own particular sensitivity; they have a direct access to their feelings that is unique to them and such strength of character can, I believe, help change the world.

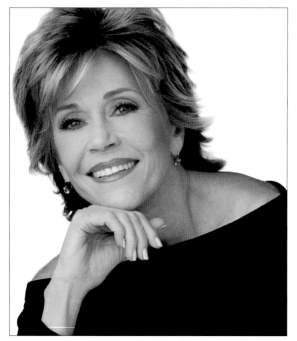

Beauty, like fashion, is a question of choice. With just one model, you can create an infinite number of photos. Working with her personality, you can invent the role that she will play in the final product. A shocking mane or straight-laced locks, infinitely long eyelashes or the reddest lips, high heels or sneakers: the possibilities are endless.

When I meet a woman for the first time, I notice her makeup but I try to see first and foremost what kind of person she is.

I love the recent films that JANE FONDA has been in. They are so full of emotion and depth! Being beautiful is not about throwing your hair around rapturously (laughing). The foundation you see here, Age Re-Perfect, was invented for mature skin — women over sixty — and I love it so much that I use it on girls who are sixteen!

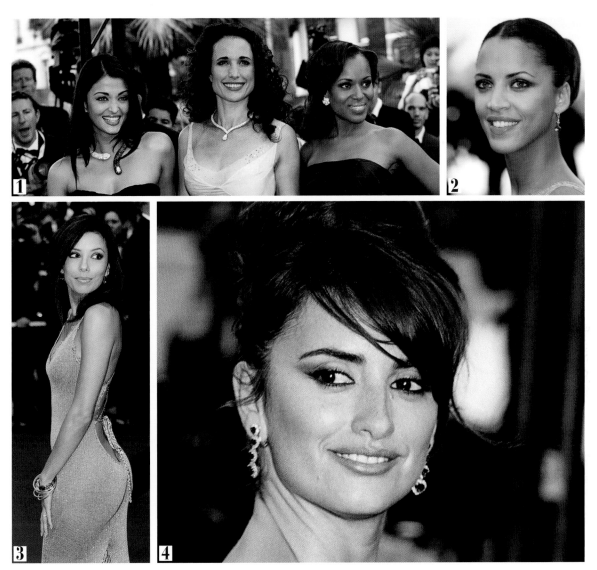

A FESTIVAL OF CHARM. 1. AISHWARYA RAI, ANDIE MACDOWELL AND KERRY WASHINGTON 2. NOÉMIE LENOIR 3. EVA LONGORIA 4. PENELOPE CRUZ. Many think, wrongly, that the beauty world is artificial, superficial: I never stop fighting against such stereotypes and always try to inject authenticity. Even if everything we do is based on technique, we really do try to bring another dimension to beauty. And doing this is all the more simple with L'Oréal Paris since our **ambassadors are not only unbelievably beautiful but they also have equally unbelievable personalities ...** They were in fact all chosen primarily for their emotional side and not just for their stunning physical traits: their look only count for about 20 per cent in our decisions. The rest lies in their manner of expressing themselves, — and that's what makes them amazing women. My mission is to help out in the fascinating crossroads that is the Cannes Film Festival. It is a huge inspiration being here, there is so much respect for artistic creation; I find it immensely moving when people jump out of their seats to clap at the end of a film ... This Festival gives great credit to the artists' work: moviegoers look beyond the "entertainment" aspect of a film and realize the immense amount of work that goes into its making. It's a miraculous thing, and what makes cinema delightful is that we see ourselves onscreen. The effect that **the actresses' beauty has on us is like a dream** — without forgetting the astonishing relationship between stars and fans and the countless declarations of love the length of the walk down the "red carpet".

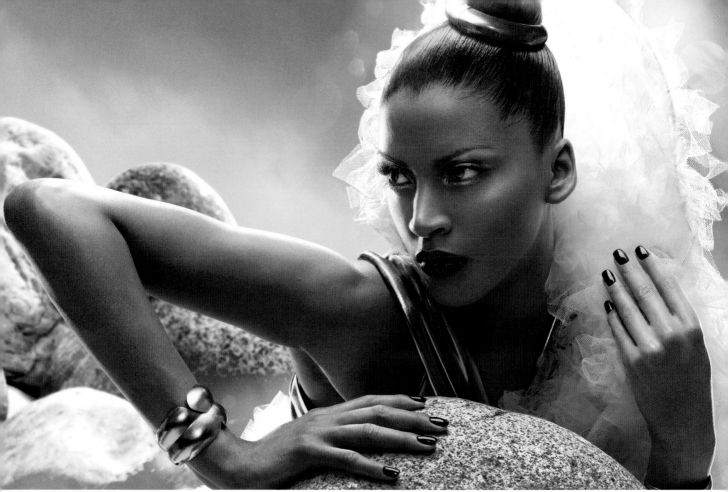

Noémie Lenoir: transfigured, surreal …

The same goes for photo shoots — I drown in the image that the model is transmitting and in the personality that she is offering to the world. Moreover, my work consists of never-ending choices to be made (OK, enough porcelain skin, let's move on!). The way you do your own hair or makeup is a choice and must be seen as such, as a way of making a statement about yourself. Beware, though, of falling into a routine. **It's important to rethink your look from time to time, to "break with tradition" and try something new** that really works for you. You don't look the same at twenty, forty, or sixty … As you grow older, you adapt and evolve as your looks change. There is nothing sad about this "beauty evolution". *Au contraire!* Listen to the advice of your beauty professionals for a new hair style, for example. I do the same thing: when I don't know what to wear I ask my stylist friends! Get your makeup done at a makeup counter: you don't have to buy a thing and if you don't like the result, you can remove it all! Above all, look around you, keep your eyes open: there is so much to take in! Get inspiration from magazines (or the pages of this book!) and you'll discover what you're naturally attracted to. It's up to you afterwards to determine what suits you best, if it's realistic (and possible!) or if it's pure fantasy. If something looks "you", go for it! Make yourself happy. There's only one way to (re)discover yourself: in a mirror, without makeup, as if you were looking at someone else. Just one rule: avoid taking a sudden dislike to what you see! Focus rather on what you like since that is what you're going to highlight. Take your eyes, for example: there are plenty of ways to play with eye

"There's only one way to (re)discover yourself: in a mirror, without makeup, as if you were looking at someone else!"

makeup! So many products are available today and you probably already spend much more on your hair than on your eyes. Take advantage of what's available. You never know, it might just change your life. Set up "beauty meetings" with your girlfriends — my mother did it; there were always women around the house getting their hair done.

What's the real secret? Light. It is fundamental in everything to do with beauty. You can do the most beautiful makeup imaginable but if you are in the wrong light, it can look awful. Mirrors aren't the most important makeup accessory, it's your lighting. That's what will show you how you'll look to others. If you say to yourself, "Oh no! that's not me" when you see yourself in a mirror during the day or in a picture, then something's gone wrong. Don't hesitate to leave the warm light of your bathroom to check your makeup in daylight or under a harsh fluorescent. It's worth a walk to the window to find the right foundation or eyeshadow!

JAMES AND HIS STARS

Some women know exactly how they want to look. **ANGELINA JOLIE** is that way: a thin, dry black line along her brows and lipstick since she doesn't like the natural color of her lips. She chose gray and I refused to use it: I prefer beige! Making up Angelina was a dream; she is so intelligent and knows what she's doing. She masters the art of her round face — eyes, lips and cheeks — by redrawing lines and creating a new structure. On the other hand, **MADONNA** is more "Do what you like!" We tried tons of new stuff together. It was intoxicating, like a "work in progress". Both approaches are enjoyable for me and I love working within strict limits. **MARILYN MANSON** also knew precisely what look he wanted, and it was grandiose! My ego is never at play, I just go with the flow of each new situation. The most wonderful compliment I ever received was from **RICHARD AVEDON**: "This kid's good!" I have had the immense privilege of working with the best photographers working today like **IRVING PENN** and **HELMUT NEWTON**. They ushered me into their world and welcomed me: it was a fabulous gift.   ▶

James's 5-minute *makeover*

FOUNDATION Always start off with a day cream and don't be shy with it. Taking good care in cleansing and moisturizing your skin is the foundation of good makeup. Next comes foundation. You'll choose one according to your skin type. I prefer foundations that cover well but that you can "work with" according to your needs. That said, new formulas are downright magical and look "real". Today's laboratories are doing incredible things. **What matters almost as much as the formula is how you apply your foundation.** Your hands must be delicate and you must learn to dose evenhandedly. A (too) common error is to apply foundation like a skin cream. Don't forget, foundation is something else entirely. Apply it in small pats on the very specific zones that need to be hidden most before delicately blending outwards on your face. A good rule of thumb is to put a small amount on your hand and to dab lightly in order to achieve a seamlessly natural look and to **avoid those oh-so disgraceful demarcation lines between your jaw and neck,** for example. Start under your eyes and then move on to all the zones you want to cover: around your nose, on your chin — all the middle areas of your face. Next, move from your cheekbones to your jaw, usually a naturally flawless zone, and blend towards your neck. I often see women doing the exact opposite, applying heavy foundation first on their cheeks and missing all the important areas altogether! **EYES** Don't shy away from **eyelash curlers — fabulous tools to discover** that I consider vital, especially if you use curving mascara! A dot of foundation on your eyelids will help prep them before applying makeup, regardless of the look you choose. Start with eyeshadow first, if you want a clearly defined eyeliner, and then apply to avoid any shadow or powder infractions. It also holds the shadow in place. On the other hand, if you're shooting for a more smudged effect, start with eyeliner and blend it into the eyeshadow that's going to cover it. **Accentuate your eyes by giving them structure** … and finish off with mascara. **CHEEKS** Use blush sparingly since your eyes are done up. **LIPS** Yet again what you'll do depends on the overall look: maybe you'll just want some gloss. Your lips will help balance out, according to your mood, a touch of shiny color that will hallmark your **final look: lipstick** always makes women look more made up. **POWDER** The perfect happy ending: that final sweep across your T-zone provides dazzling confirmation that your makeup took only five minutes to apply — from cream to powder including eyes, lips and cheeks!

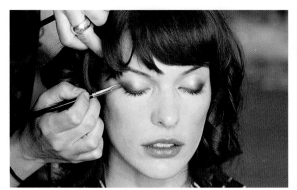
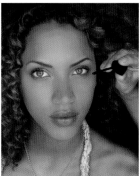
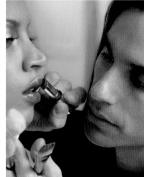

From Milla's eyelids to Noémie's lips, James applies the same loving attention to detail.

Laetitia, the most vibrant of canvases, under James's masterful brush stroke.

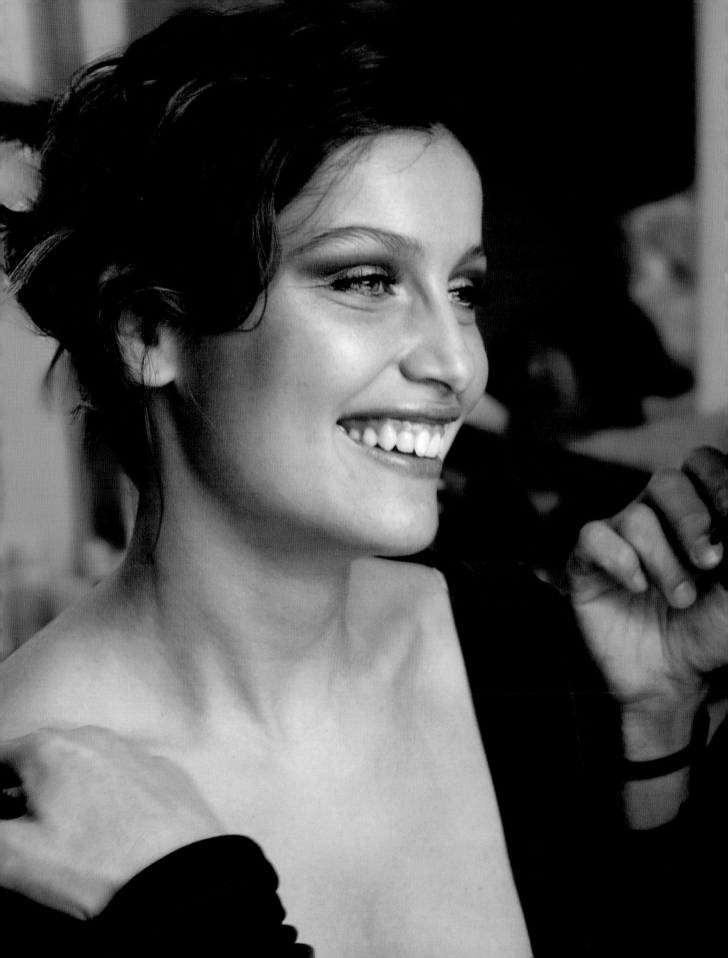

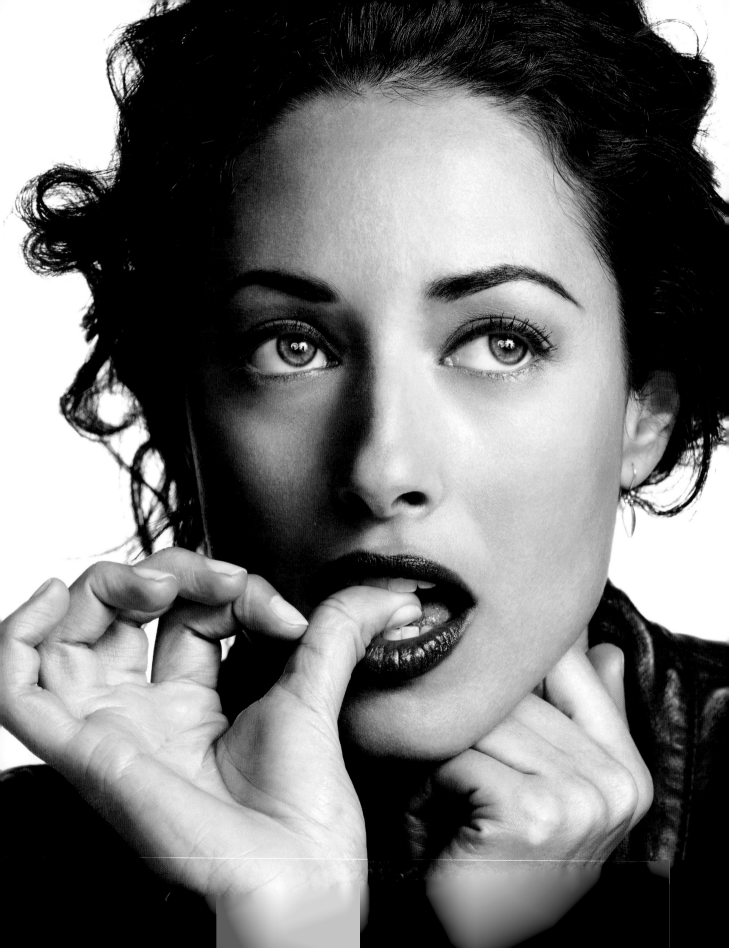

Bobbi Brown
Founder and C.E.O. of Bobbi Brown Cosmetics

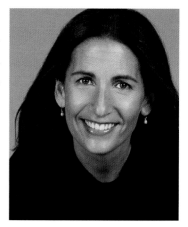

Hailed as the "Princess of the Palette" by the American press, Bobbi Brown is one of a kind. Flaunting her unique "feel good" approach to beauty, she holds her own in the highly select club of celebrity makeup artists. Her motto? "Be who you are." And her mission: help every woman reclaim her own beauty.

"All I want is for my makeup to make women happy!"

I don't think that I'm particularly different, I simply think that I am more in tune with ordinary women; I see myself in every one. It's a little harder with top models whose glamorously sublime pictures in the magazines aren't necessarily anchored in real life, where you just want to look pretty and bring out the best in yourself, starting over every morning with what you've got. That type of 'real life' is second-nature to me — and I'd love for that to be the case for all women! That's what I want to get across to women everywhere. 'Beautiful' doesn't mean looking younger than you are, it just means looking great!

It's easy to think that beauty starts with your eyes or your mouth. That's wrong: the first ingredient of beauty is skin. Whether you have wrinkles or are barely twenty, if you can achieve a seamless complexion without looking 'made up', then you have what it takes. After all, it's their dreamlike skin that makes the top models so stunning … But then again, at thirteen anything is possible!

French women are so confident and in touch with themselves. They are secure in their own unique seductiveness. But I still find it strange that you never see women over the age of thirty in the magazines. You can be inspired by the models but one doesn't necessarily identify with them. **You want to know my approach to being yourself? Don't ever compare yourself to anyone. It's fine to admire but not to compete. You'll only wind up losing!"**

The color chocolate, a delicious concoction by Bobbi Brown.

"There's always a way to be your best you."

As a woman, I've always known what women wanted to look like, even top models. It is important to me that my products make women happy. That's rare in this business — most makeup artists don't care. For me, what matters is that women feel attractive, model or not. If I were working a show and the girls asked for makeup remover as soon as they stepped off the podium, I'd take it as an insult.

At twenty you're sublime, but you don't know it. When I was that age, thrown into the high-fashion world fresh from my native Midwest, I didn't have the slightest idea.

You never think you've "made it", and I've only felt that way for the past four years or so. **The difference? I don't try anymore to be something. I just am.**

It's an unbelievably comfortable feeling, and people are always telling me how good I look, how refreshed, even at parties where I'm hanging around in jeans hobnobbing with top models (cheating a little with heels since I'm so short!).

On the other hand, if you try to be something you're not, it will never work.

Being yourself means taking hold of everything you can that will make you feel (and look) your best. And when being true to yourself, whatever the situation, there is always a way to be at your best — thanks to makeup!

Of course makeup is only part of a bigger package: taking care of yourself means eating well, drinking plenty of water — without forgetting that organic vegetables or other health foods can go well with a good glass of wine (for example, I think Chianti, works perfectly with olive oil, dark chocolate and green tea) — and not smoking. Let's not forget about choosing the right clothes, including the right underwear (it's no use trying to feel great if they're not practical!).

And don't forget, makeup is not a question of what's trendy, but of personal style. You can find one that's right for you at any age! We've understood that in the cosmetics industry: when we've developed the products that are right for you, we don't change them. That's the reasoning behind the permanence of our trademark lines.

Call a spade a spade: I'm still makeup artist, and I love working on fashion shoots, brushing shoulders with the stars, and experimenting on them in the heat of the moment — too much, too bright — and seeing that they're still sublime.

All the same, when I see a woman for the first time, I see the person, not the makeup she's wearing. And I'm happy for that or else I'd go crazy! What I do notice on the other hand is when makeup is too brutal or too played-up. Within moments of seeing a face for the first time I know what it needs. My job, after all, is training makeup professionals!

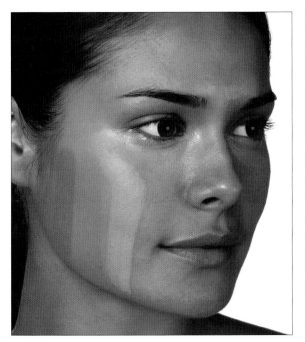
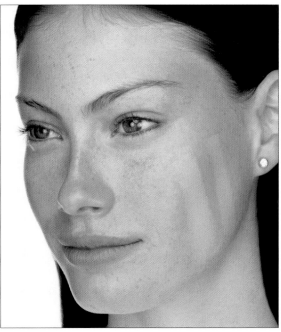

A TRICK TO FINDING THE PERFECT FOUNDATION. Try a stick, it's easier for testing: apply three different shades on your lower cheek, and pat the three of them to find the right shade for you: choose the one that you can barely see, that's neither oily or yellow (and pick concealer one shade lighter).

Bobbi's *touch* in ten easy steps

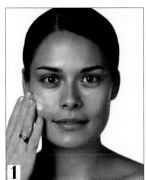
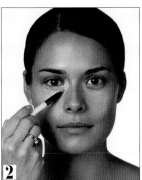
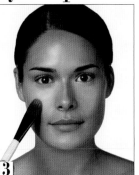
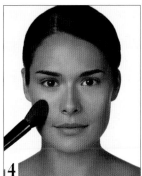

COMPLEXION. 1. Moisturizing base: polymers help to create a healthy backdrop. City girls' dry skin is particularly resistant to any makeup: if your skin is not correctly treated first, nothing will stick! Smooth out around you eyes with a specialized moisturizer before applying your concealer (so that it holds fast better). 2. Applying corrector with a brush both neutralizes the shadows under your eyes and perks up your face. For bluish shadows under your eyes, use a rosy color. To protect the creamy base, dab gently up to the lash line and around your whole eye. 3. Use a brush to apply a generous amount of under-eye concealer (too much comes out if you use your fingers). Trace a flat contour around your eyebrows and gently wipe off any excess with your finger.

Bobbi's *touch* in ten easy steps

4. **FOUNDATION:** Brushes allow for a lighter finish but you have more control using your fingers. Use yellow undertones and never rose-toned ones. Massage and powder then remove excess with a large brush — for normal to oily skin that tends to shine. Lightly veil the concealer with a blender brush. You can also use matte tanning powder (test on your shoulders or forearm) for a "sun-kissed" look. Blush, too, is possible: while smiling, accentuate your cheekbones through an outward and downward movement to hit the zones where you naturally blush.

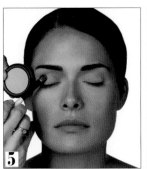 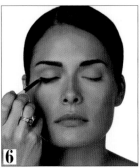 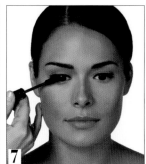 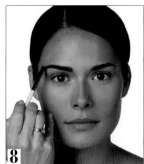

EYES 5. For basic makeup: a brush-applied matte color spread on your eyelid (tap away any excess). For a more sophisticated look: apply shadow onto the brush and then press on your hand so that the product penetrates deeply — and correct with a blender brush and a cotton swab. Accentuate the effect with a darker shadow around the eye contours, either dry or mixed with water. 6. Trace the baseline of your eye with an eyeliner pencil. Highlight only by filling in above the lash line and don't try to modify its shape. Lightly pull your eyelid and fill in the roots of eyelashes. Gel eyeliner, does not run, is water-resistant and easy to use. What's more, it glides on practically on its own. It provides a guaranteed optical illusion like a second set of lashes, sober and elegant at the same time. 7. Mascara: start from the roots and turn the brush as you pull it, like you would while drying your hair. Use a zigzag movement to create volume and thicken. 8. Don't forget your eyebrows: use eyebrow mascara that's the natural color of your hair (or clear) for thicker brows, and a bevelled-edge brush for thinner ones.

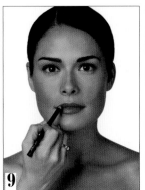 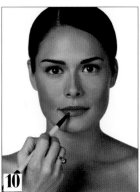

LIPS 9. After lipstick application, use your lip liner for blending while maintaining a natural appeal. 10. Gloss will give your lips a smooth and softly radiant look. You can mix iridescent pinks with a matte tone. And why not a touch of lilac-infused gloss in the middle of your lips?

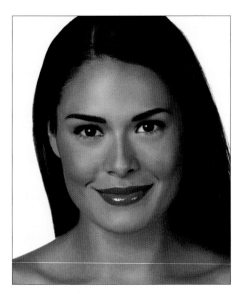

Manda as seen through Bobbi's eyes.

"Why have your eyelids redone? Just add some eyeliner."

When people talk about "revolutions" in the cosmetics industry, it's much more a question of common sense than "technology" (that's just marketing jargon): what matters are formulas. The ones that sell best are thick and neither oily nor too dry. Even if no cream definitively erases wrinkles today, it is true that advances in technology have given us the possibility to add sunscreen to it. Regardless, the real key is effective moisturizing. I am particularly proud of my Extra Moisturizing Balm — I feel the difference when I put it on only one part of my face.

How did I invent my eyeliner gel? You should know I'm a very practical person. That day, I was in Colorado for a photo shoot (it was *my* picture being taken!) and, rifling through my bag, I realized I'd forgotten my eyeliner. I only had black mascara and I used it to line my eyes and — surprise! — it held all day. I immediately called my office and said, "We're going to invent the first eyeliner that is ready for the long haul." That is how I work. Feeling good at any age means being in control: a little effort on your hair and makeup … I've never wanted to have my eyelids redone — all you need to do is add more eyeliner! Compulsive cosmetic surgery makes me sick: women never look younger or more beautiful; they just look like they've had something done. The more you're worried about your body, the more it shows on your face.

BOBBI AND HER STARS

As far as celebrities go, I adore Jodie Foster: she's so beautiful, so kind, simple … normal, in a word. I gave her a "French actress" look that I really like, a little jumbled, based all in navy blue … I also made up Meryl Streep. But the most beautiful woman I have ever worked on was Brooke Shields: she was fourteen at the time, and breathtaking. That skin, those lips, those eyes! That was my favorite photo shoot.

EXPRESS MAKEUP TIPS

AND SHE'S OFF! Five minutes before leaving the house … If you're blonde with fair skin, don't go out without mascara. Similarly, a darker-skinned brunette can not do without her lipstick. **MY ORDER: #1:** Hydrating base **#2:** foundation **#3:** blush **#4:** eyeliner. Lips last: you can always touch up with a bit of gloss while stopping in front of a store window. **My secret weapon:** a small, all-in-one makeup kit, with six compartments: correcting cream, three shades of concealer, foundation, a bright blush for my cheeks and my favorite lipstick.

"Even in the evening, there's no need for exaggeration: I'm more about nuances and hints than overstatement."

GOOD EVENING MAKEUP KIT!

The difference between daytime and evening makeup is not as dramatic as you might think. Shinier lipstick and black rather than brown for the eyes usually suffice. Some women opt for more flashy, sparkly effects. I'm more about hints and nuances than overstatement.

BOBBI'S FAVORITE TRICKS

FOUNDATION There's only one reason to wear it: for a seamless complexion. To ensure that you have the right color, test a little on the side of your face, above your jaw. Be careful: the skin on your face is often lighter than on the rest of the body. Depending on the occasion, you can choose a clear foundation or a bronzing powder.

EYEBROWS should be in harmony with your face. If your facial features are pronounced, your brows should be too. If your face is more delicate, your eyebrow lines should be accordingly lighter. But they should always remain natural. Luckily we're no longer living in the age of brow massacres: waxed, plucked to death or even shaved — they never grew back!

SUN I'm one of the rare makeup artists to believe that sun brings out women's natural beauty. And protecting your skin (with maximum SPF facial sunscreen) still allows for a pretty tan!

BLUSH What's the right color? The one that appears when you pinch your cheeks.

EYES To look as natural as can be, mascara should be as dark as possible. I like it black, very black, and rich. Most women put too much importance on eyeshadow. I believe it should come after eyebrows, eyeliner and mascara: those three are the real key. You must buy shadow in just the right color and it should require no extra work: it is very difficult to subdue a very dark eyeshadow.

LIPS The ideal lipstick color is the one that complements the natural color of your lower lip: if it blends well there, you can be sure it works. You can go lighter or brighter, but I wouldn't recommend going darker: it can age you and doesn't look as good.

HOLD IT! Mixing your makeup (eyeliner + powder, foundation + powder) multiplies durability tenfold • remove any oily residue before doing your eyelids • using two blushes will make it look like you've just put it on: use a natural shade and a slighter lighter one on top and it will last at least half the day • don't forget to reapply concealer in the middle of the day.

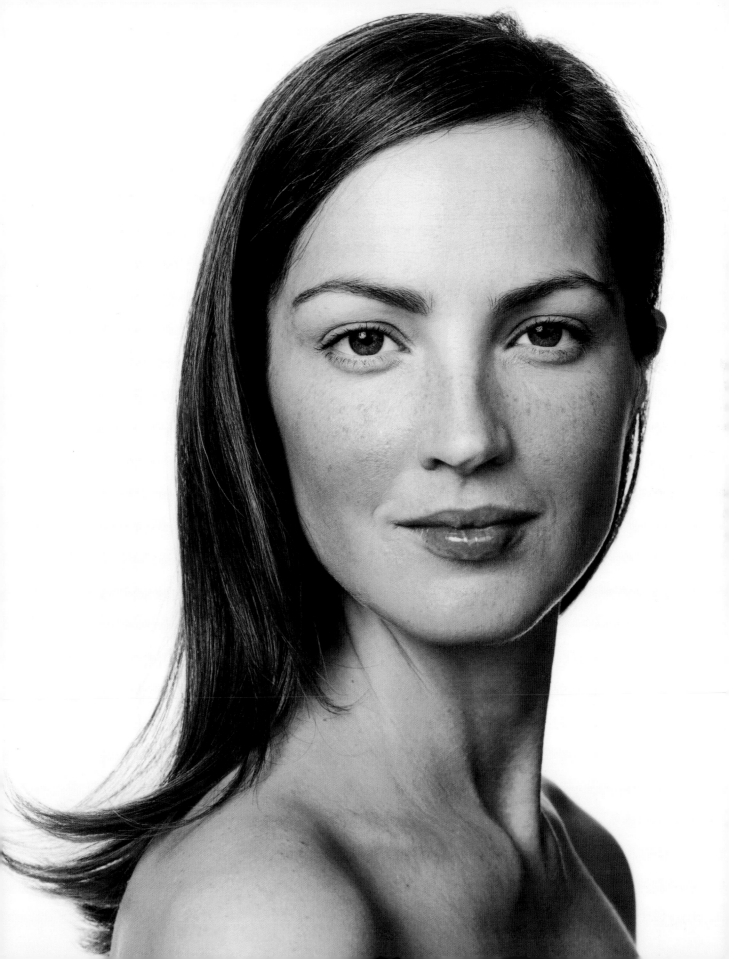

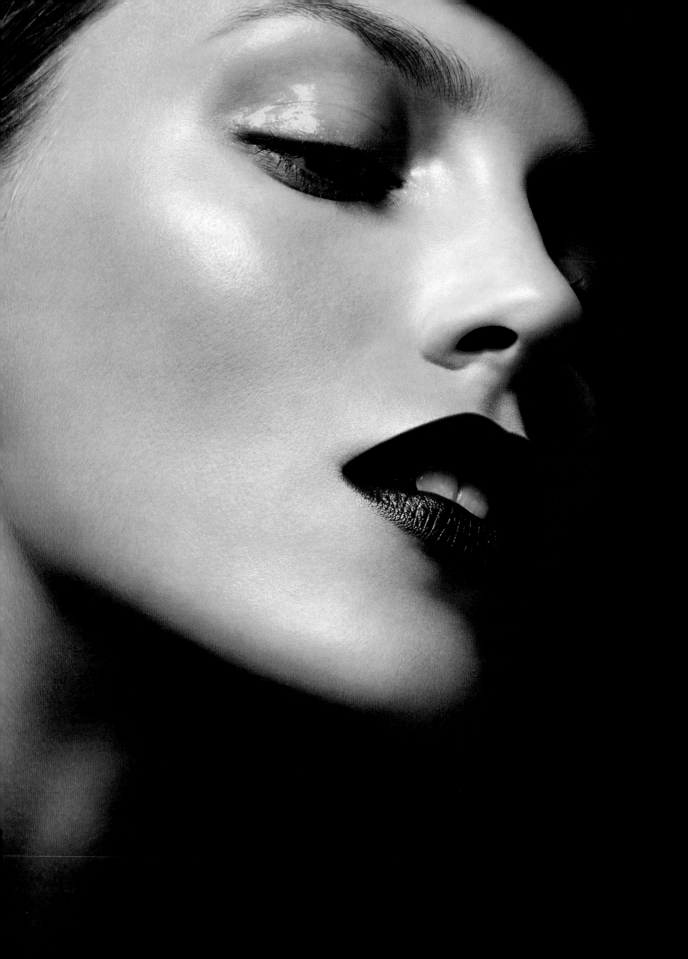

Giorgio Armani
Cosmetics

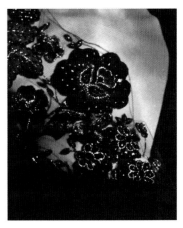

"Like fashion, makeup is an expression of femininity. It should be easy to apply yet still bring some element of fantasy." The Italian fashion designer goes from clothes to makeup with the same taste for airy materials and purity of color …

"There is **nothing** in the world more **sensual** than **swathing** a body in fabric and wrapping a **face** in a veil of **smooth textures**."

Giorgio Armani

Makeup according to Armani? It's a wardrobe for the face that you pick according to your mood. The Italian designer's entire philosophy is in that one sentence, in a spirit of luxury and freedom: **'To be elegant is not to be noticed. It is to be unforgettable …'** Where to start? Every woman has her own approach to beauty. She wants to 'be beautiful', and that's more fundamental than highlighting her eyes or lips. Clients' expectations from the cosmetics industry have greatly changed. They're looking for professional-quality tools and techniques all in radiance and lightness that are available to them on a day-to-day basis. No masks or rigid effects; it's all about luminous textures and a 'no makeup' effect. The more made up you are, the more natural you should appear; but it's a very meticulous 'natural'. More than just makeup, Armani's products are an extension of his clothing: pure and airy textures enclosing ultra-fine pigments that melt beautifully into the skin, available in an array of Mediterranean shades, soft monochromes and subtle harmonies, containing nothing but the noblest ingredients. An exclusive technology (Micro-Fil™) from the clothing industry affords translucent colors and ultra-smooth textures that you can endlessly superimpose. In this way, blush will reignite the pink of your cheeks after a morning run in chilly weather. The prettiest illustration of what Giorgio Armani hopes to offer women is a palette that 'will allow them to express the myriad nuances of their emotions'."

THE ART OF A NATURALLY LUMNIOUS COMPLEXION

Laurent Martin, Face Designer, Giorgio Armani Cosmetics

MAGNIFY (BASE MAKEUP — FOUNDATION — CONCEALER)

1. On perfectly clean and moisturized skin, use base to get a flawless complexion: apply a thin layer with your fingertips, spreading from the center of the face outwards. With your hand cupped in a half-circle, touch up with light pressure along the contours of your face, the sides of your nose and your jaw: your facial traits will be perfectly blended. **2.** Brush techniques (see page 189). **3.** To hide redness and small imperfections as well as bags, pimples or other signs of fatigue, apply concealer to the outer and inner corners of your eye and around the edges of your nose. With the help of a highlighting brush, apply a small amount to problem areas and dab lightly with your fingertips so that the texture blends impeccably with your foundation.

ILLUMINATE (LIQUID LUMINIZER — POWDER)

4. As soon as you attract light to a particular spot on your face, you "reveal" it by adding volume through optical illusion. According to your mood, all combinations are possible: nuances afforded by luminizers are true gems. These products will create a radiant glow and embellish your most prominent facial traits — cheeks, forehead, inner eye corner, upper cheekbone and under the eyebrow arch. **5.** Micro-Fil™ Loose Powder envelops your face in a radiant veil and reduces shine. Apply the powder liberally with a brush on the face's middle zone for a discreet and naturally luminous glow. For a more sophisticated look, apply the powder to your whole face as well as on your neck and shoulders.

SHAPE AND CURVE (LUMINIZING LIQUID — BLUSH AND BRONZING POWDER)

6. Creating depth means creating shadows and redesigning the contours of your face. Depending on the look you want, use copper- or pink-toned luminizing formulas. Apply below your cheekbones to make them stand out, on your temples, along your jaw line and on the sides and tip of your nose to refine its volume. Use one dose of product for each zone and reapply as necessary. **7.** The final

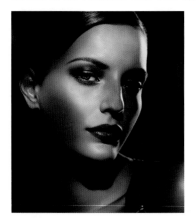

touch for a flawless complexion: sheer blush for a velvety finish or cream blush for a "no makeup" look. Apply in small dabs to your face then blend with a brush. For a breezy look, apply on your cheeks or under your cheekbones for glowing, fresh-faced feel. **8.** Finally, if you're looking for a sophisticated and glamorous finish, bronzing powder can be swept on the center of your cheeks and the tip of your nose, the first places that natural sunlight would hit your face.

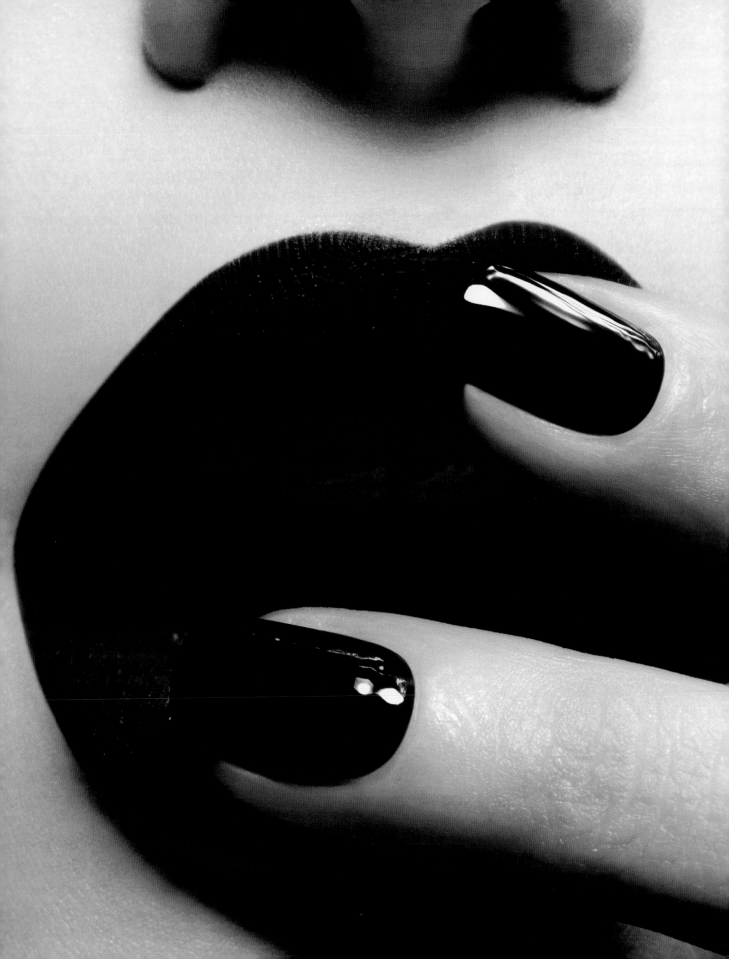

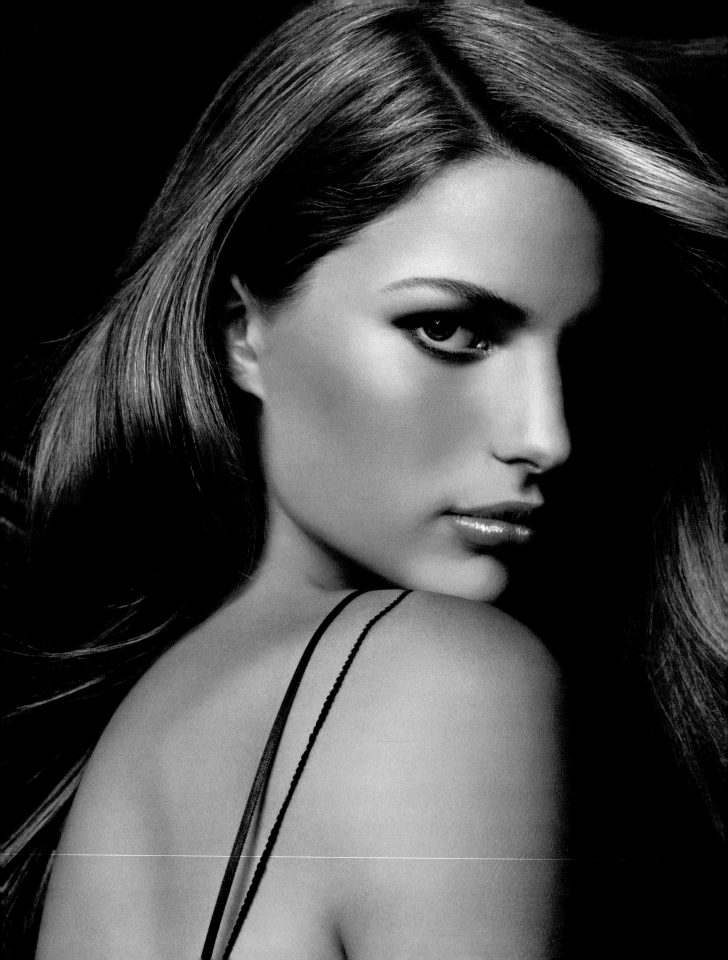

"My work consists not in superfluous add-ons but rather in purifying basics. Less is more."

Giorgio Armani

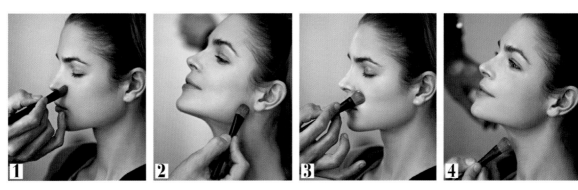

COMPLEXION: Brush techniques. 1. Before applying foundation, warm the product up on the back of your hand with a foundation brush. Dot a small quantity of product on the tip of your brush. This technique allows you to modulate the intensity of your makeup according to the desired final product. Always start in the center of your face and work outwards. 2. Continue with broad and regular movements and spread the product outwards with upward movements towards your hairline. 3. Always work with a gentle foundation brush when dealing with sensitive spots where redness can develop such as the sides of your nose, the outer corner of your eye and the corners of your lips. 4. Finish off with circular movements of the foundation brush from your jawline down to your neck.

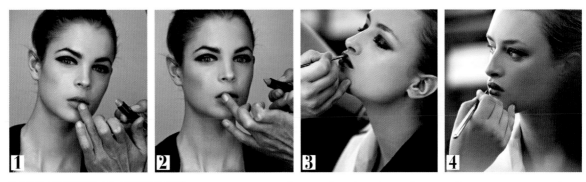

LIPS: NATURAL EFFECTS: 1. Prep your lips first with a clear lipstick 0: opt for a transparent, shiny shade in beige or pink and apply with your finger. 2. End with your upper lip while tapping the middle of your lip for a "plumper" finish. 3. For glamorous lips, prep them first with clear lipstick 0 and redefine the contours of your lips with a smooth silk lip pencil 4 for perfect lines. Blend the interior of your lips with a lip brush then apply ArmaniSilk 10 lipstick, our signature red, still using your lip brush. 4. For an ultra-glamorous and sparkling finish, apply a glittery top coat in the middle of your lips. Sensual lips for a sophisticated finish …

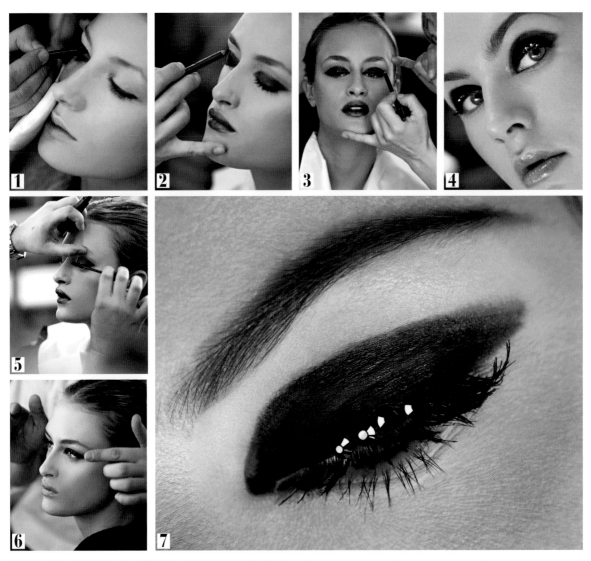

EYE GRAPHIC: BACKSTAGE IN MAKEUP 1. Use a smooth silk eye pencil to sketch a line along your lashes. Define your workspace by drawing a line in the crease of your eyelid. 2. Color in the entire eyelid up to the crease with the same pencil. For added sparkle, extend along to the outer corner of your eye. 3. For greater depth, apply your eyeshadow as a fixer on top of the eyeliner. Use an eyeshadow brush and dot the product on lightly from the inside out for a seamless finish. 4. Using your silky smooth lip pencil, highlight the crease of your eyelid by extending color from the inner corner to the outer corner of your eye. With the help of an eye contour brush, use to-and-fro movements to blend the pencil. 5. For a captivating gaze, use star lash mascara, placing the curved end of the brush to the roots covering the whole lash. Repeat, using the other end of the contoured brush to add volume. 6. To bring life to the corners of your eye, set the makeup by tapping with the flat of your fingertip. 7. Black crystals glued in the center of fake eyelashes are the ultimate final touch for sparkling sophistication.

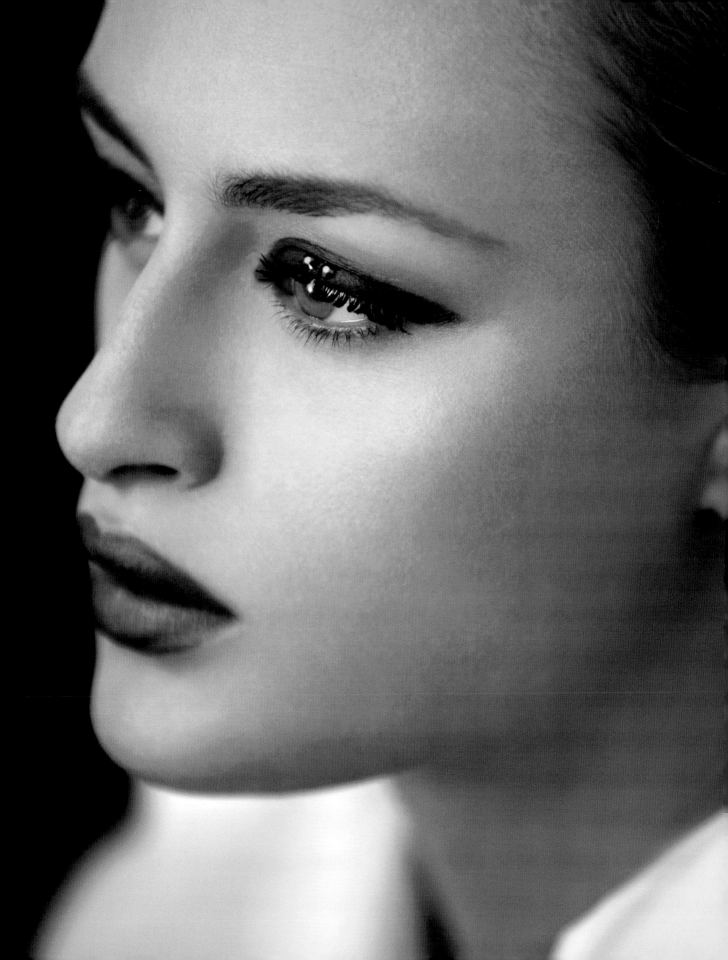

MAKEUP ARTISTS' TRADE SECRETS

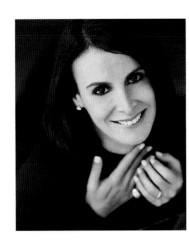

Terry
Founder of by Terry

A true star in the fashion industry, Terry's line is firmly implanted in the beauty market and has inspired the greatest haute couture designers. She stands resolutely against standardization of the industry and is for individualization and the integrity of creativity.

"**Makeup** today is more about **polishing** your **natural beauty** rather than pseudo-**perfection**."

What's modernity? It's the anti-effect: **the ultimate art of being natural.** A bare face with a few brilliant details, **plump lips**, spontaneous beauty … Getting it just right is the absolute key. Accentuate light that is there naturally before trying to add more. I see no need for a foundation promising a supposedly flawless complexion. Today, women are using more and more makeup, and it shows less and less. No more masks: it's about showcasing what you've already got and specific gestures to plump up, conceal or **reveal your natural beauty**. Makeup today is more about polishing your natural beauty rather than pseudo-perfection according to randomly defined rules of what's beautiful. Everyone has natural beauty, and my philosophy is to respect and work with it. What I find interesting is when a woman who believes herself all-too ordinary looks in the mirror and suddenly finds herself scintillating. Being attentive to women helps me to see that spark and make them feel less guilty. Every woman has a right — now, more than ever — to be a little narcissistic.

INTERESTED IN A STUDIO SECRET?

I used to mix three products (foundation, hydrating cream and smoothing gel) and place it around eyes and on necks: it gave immediate freshness. Using a brush, delicately apply the mixture to your eye area, hollow of your chin, contour of your lips and the sides of our nose.

Terry's wildly rich palette, showcased here is like a case full of dream-colored jewels.

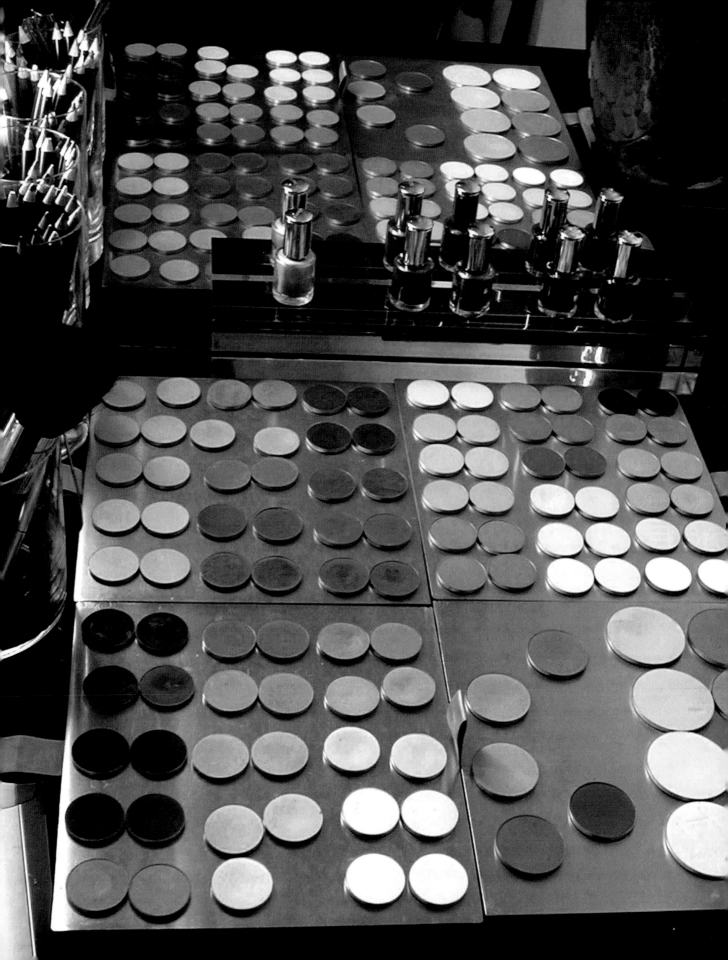

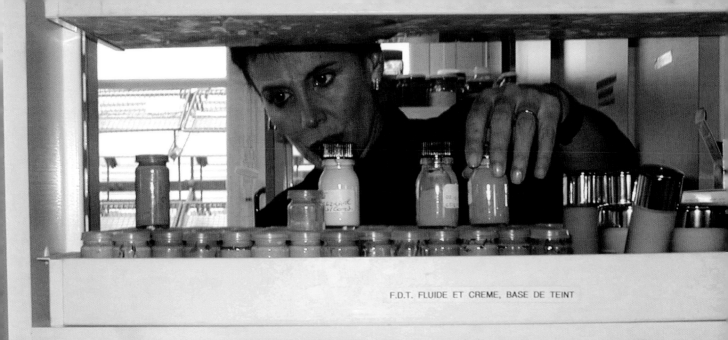

F.D.T. FLUIDE ET CREME, BASE DE TEINT

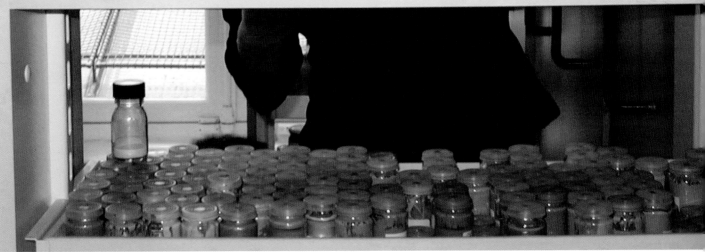

Terry in her secret laboratory.

Blend with your fingertips and you'll look like you've had a **full night's sleep**. What I want to create are concrete, no-nonsense products that facilitate women's lives. I've developed transparent formulas that respect your skin while correcting it. Research and technology give rise to modern miracles like faux-white pigments and illusion-creating coverage. That glow, that brilliance is also about color: transparent lip gloss or a true pink blush over a tan; a turquoise kohl pencil that creates mysterious eyes or eyeshadow that makes the color of your eyes pop …

You must feel good about yourself before trying to seduce others. Down with stereotypes. The fashion industry has educated people: there are fewer catastrophes with beauty victims than with fashion victims! It's about controlled freedom and you have to find your own way. You'll never be a professional so don't try to become an at-home makeup artist. I'll give you a remote control with two buttons: 'on' and 'off'. I'll deal with making it work. You just enjoy it!"

"There are fewer catastrophes with beauty victims than with fashion victims!"

TERRY'S TOUCH, LIVE FROM HER STUDIO

COMPLEXION My primary obsession is radiance! After the development of Color Skin Enhancer — veritable hours of sleep in a jar — my research team perfected a revolutionary formula enclosed in a gifted little brush called Light-Expert Foundation Brush: it knows how to exfoliate! Its feather-light texture, eye-defying coverage and innovative application make it the perfect foundation for every occasion. Even the clumsiest women will be proud of themselves. It comes in four zero-risk shades that suit virtually every skin tone.

Directions Click and dab the brush over areas needing light — under your eyes, on the tip of your chin, your cheekbones, forehead, and the sides of your nose. Blend with the brush and you have instant radiance. Try it: you can't go wrong!

CHEEKS A little pink on your cheeks is like a breath of fresh air. It raises your spirits and perks up your face. For a long time blush was controversial but I have always believed in it and used it. It gives you guaranteed freshness and suits everyone: utterly sublime on darker tones and delicate on fairer complexions.

EYES I like to set eyes against a dark backdrop like a jeweller sets a precious stone. Sometimes I blend my Powder Eye Shadow onto my Blackstar makeup to give greater intensity and durability. And mascara is a must! Generously cover the whole lash from root to tip. For the clumsy ones among you, I have a sure-fire tip for removing excess.

Directions Dip a cotton swab in my Color Skin Enhancer — Rose Light #2 or Apricot #5. Roll and blend on the back of your hand. When used as a "corrector", it will dissolve mistakes without removing your makeup.

LIPS If your eye makeup is really pronounced, I would aim for more natural lips: hydrate and color with my Laque de Rose. Every woman will find her own color in keeping with her mood. If your eyes are more sober then you can really shoot for the stars with your lips: plump them up with lipliner and blend with a brush. I use a brush to apply my Rouge Delectation. I prefer straightforward colors like Naughty Raspberry #13, Plum Marmalade #15 or Red Caramel #1.

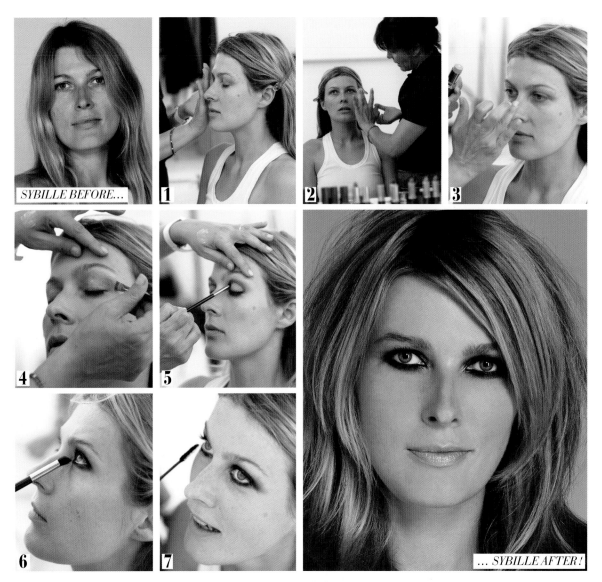

SYBILLE BEFORE…

1

2

3

4

5

6

7

… SYBILLE AFTER!

SYBILLE, 38 YEARS OLD, BEAUTY AU NATURAL … 1. Sybille's skin has been thoroughly hydrated with my Hydra-Replenishing Cream. 2. Since her face is lacking radiance, I generously applied Color Skin Enhancer Apricot #5 that will create light-plays across her face. 3. For a naturally flawless complexion, I used a Densiliss Stick Skin Glow Foundation Pale Amber #5 on her prominent features and blended with my fingertips. This is an ideal product for hiding all blemishes and imperfections. 4. I've evened out her eyelids with Powder Eye Shadow Misty Mauve #15. 5. With the help of a Dôme Brush 2, I've tuned the crease with Powder Eye Shadow Black Tulip #46: it's the ideal color for highlighting blue eyes. 6. I've redrawn Sybille's lower eye with the same powder and Precision Brush #4, close to the roots, so that Sybille's gaze is set in a ribbon of sober and velvety color. 7. Her lower eyelashes are treated to Silky Conditioning Mascara to enlarge her eyes **… AND REINVENTED BY TERRY.** The contours of her face completely redefined, Sybille has reclaimed radiant skin. To attract attention to the rest of her face — and to avoid overdoing it — I've left her lips virtually untouched.

PATTY, 51 YEARS OLD, BEAUTY AU NATURAL … 1. and 2. Patty's skin enjoyed a long massage with my deep-cleansing Purifying Serenity Cream. Her natural glow is already starting to emerge … 3. Patty didn't want anything too heavy so I applied Perfecting Glow Foundation Advanced Radiant Beige #3 with my brush. It's a fluid foundation that finishes off powdery, matte and translucent. I top it off with Loose Powder Apricot #5. 4. A pea-sized drop of liquid blush is applied transparently to the cheeks. 5. Here I add a thin line of Blackstar Black Emerald #3 to outline the eye and then blend it with a brush for a more natural look. I do the same work on the lower eyelid but with Venetian Brown #7 Silky Eye Shadow. 6. Patty's eyelashes are covered in Silky Conditioning Mascara. 7. After a Baume de Rose massage, Patty's lips are nourished and plumped and excess is wiped away with a tissue. Rouge Delectation Exquisite Cherry #14 brushed on her lips gives a fruity radiance with subtle satin sheen … **AND REINVENTED BY TERRY.** Patty has been literally transformed. She has gained freshness and spontaneity. Her blue eyes stand out and her "forbidden fruit" lips are unquestionably glamorous.

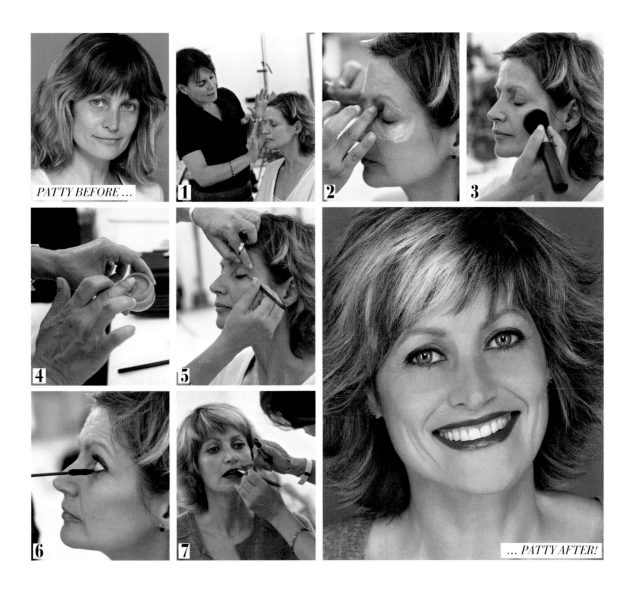

PATTY BEFORE …

1

2

3

4

5

6

7

… PATTY AFTER!

7 big night

WHEN YOU WANT TO GO WILD

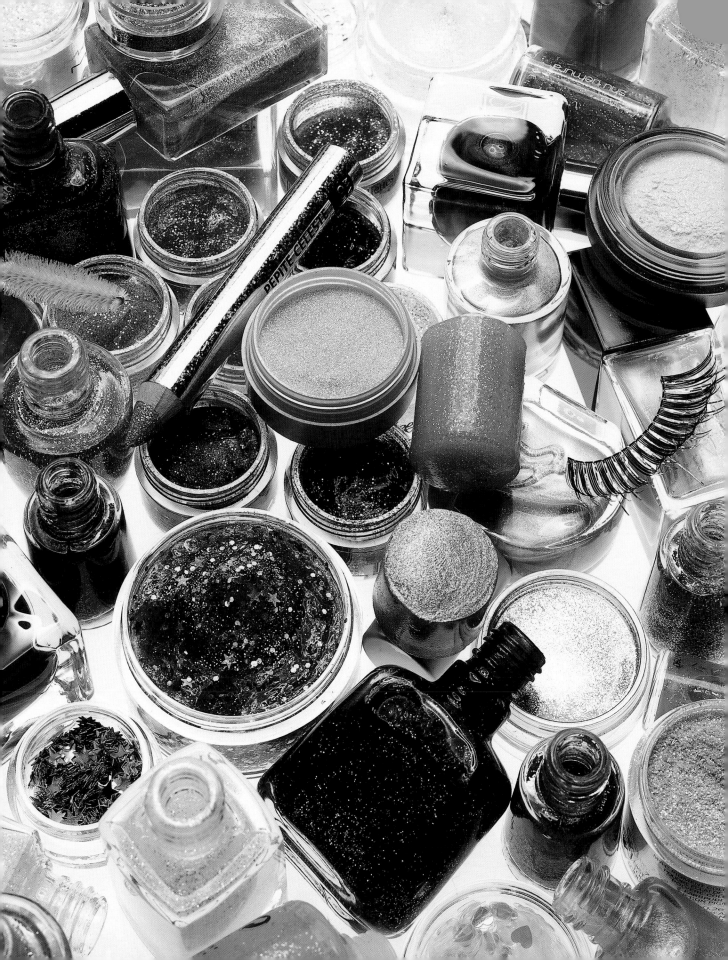

Sly panther or demure fawn: the night was meant for extremes.

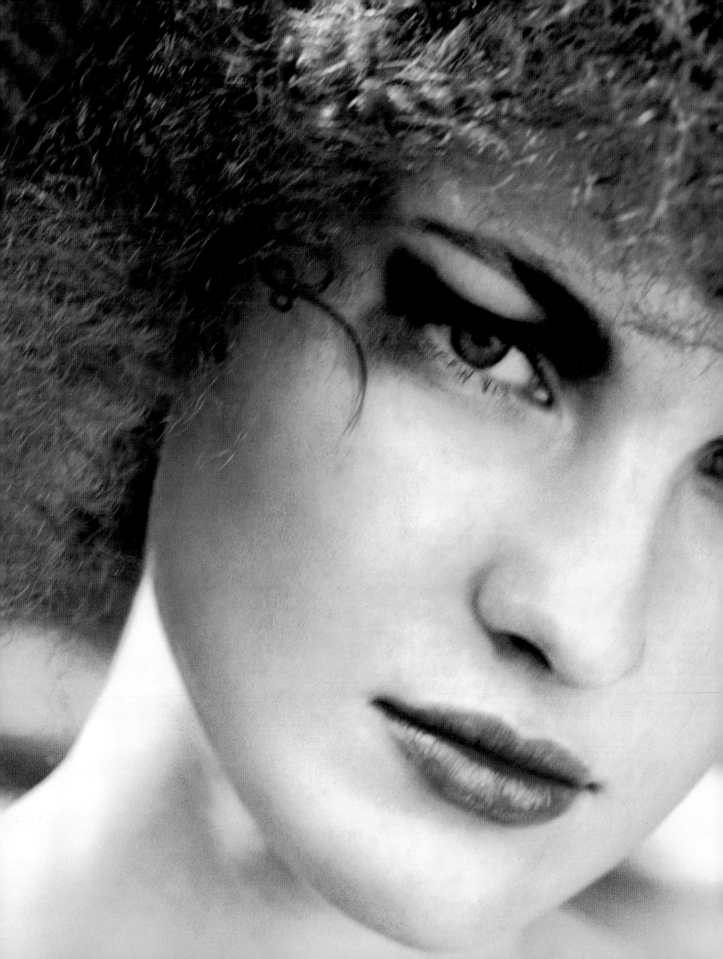

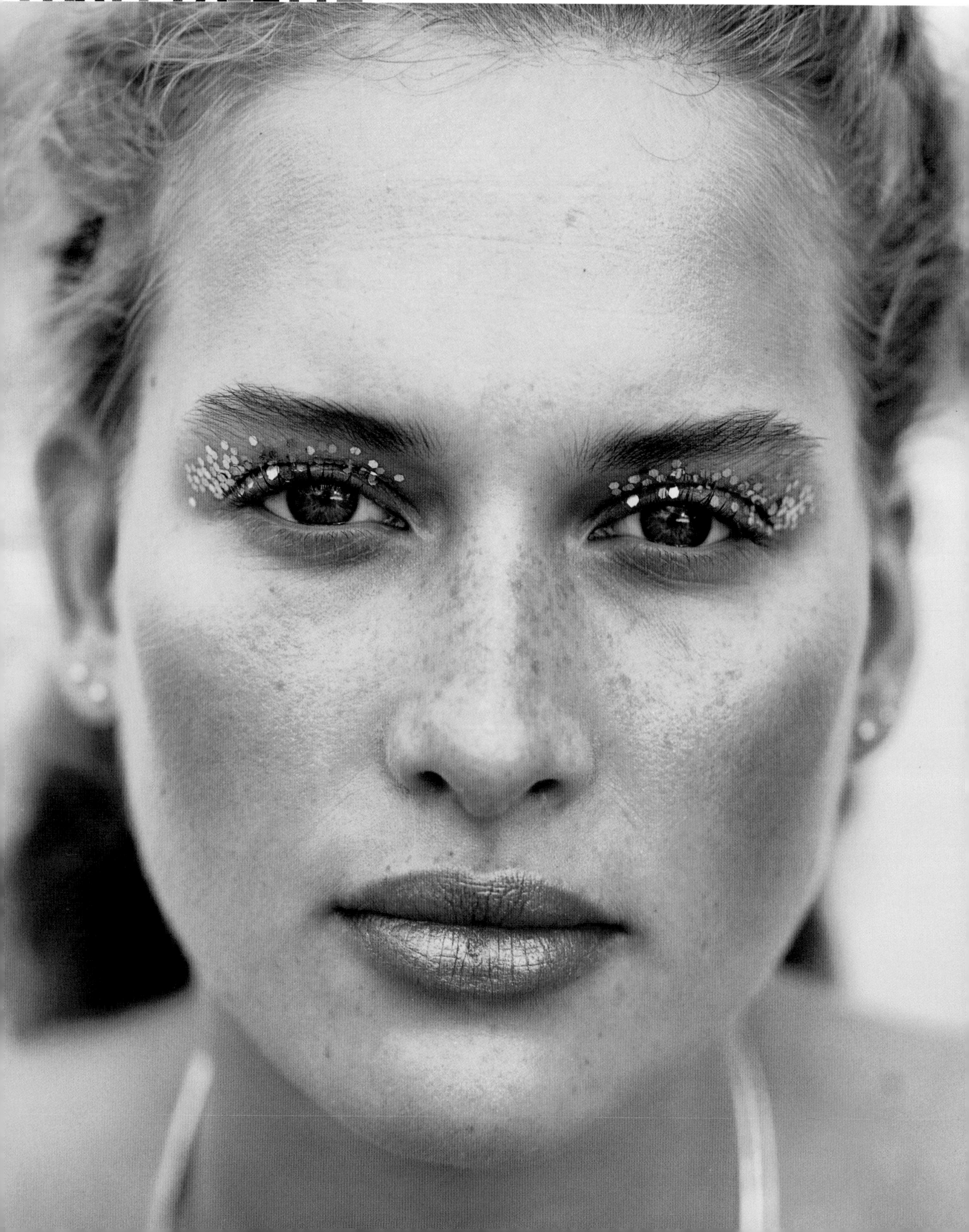

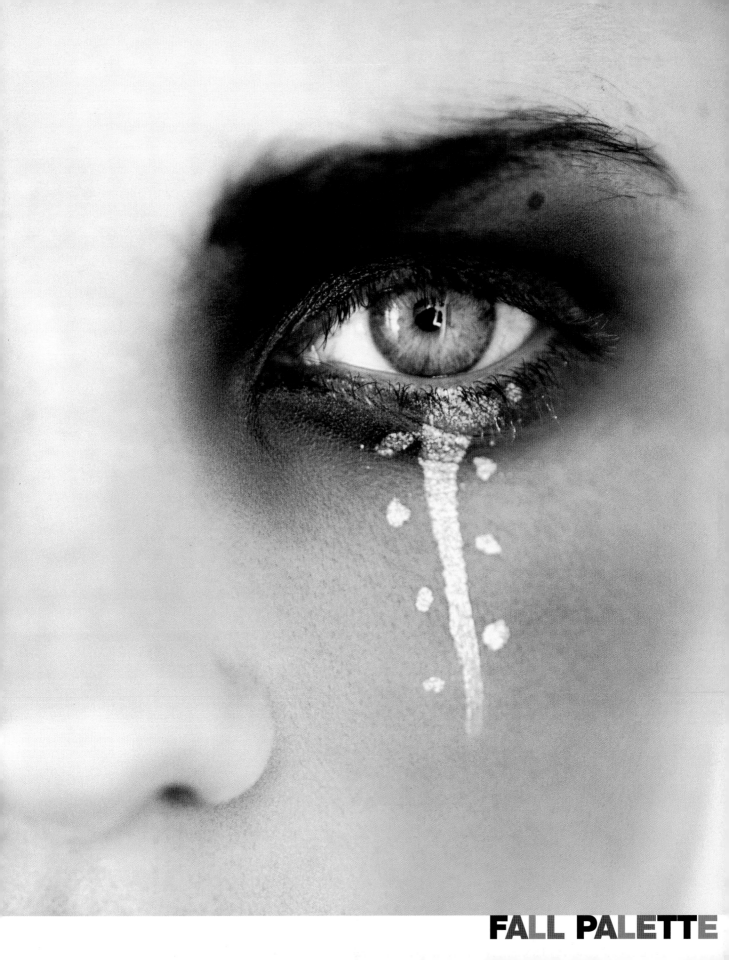

FALL PALETTE

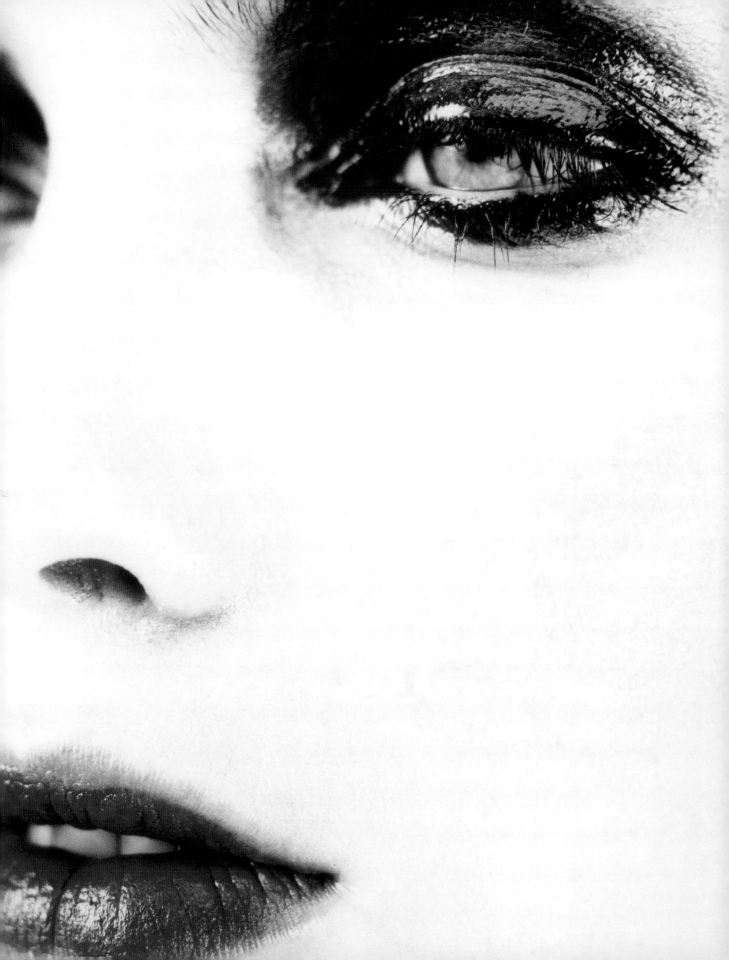

Dark
— extreme —
mysterious
black sleek
and chic …

GLITTERY GO-OUT LOOKS

Special Effects: Glitter and lights and everything nice

It's party time! Celebrate! Senses, colors, textures: Give your face an intoxicating look for that special night out.

GLITTER AND MYSTIFYING COLOR will make you gorgeous in the most unexpected ways. Shoulder-to-shoulder, above the strap of your heels, on your hairline or above your cheekbone: don't be afraid to sparkle! Powder it on lightly after applying some essential oils — or on top of freshly-applied gloss.

LIQUID GOLD a simple streak of gold or silver eyeliner will reorient your look completely. Don't overdo it: you want that unmistakable and defining detail, not to look like a Christmas tree! With a well-chosen colored mascara over a black kohl base on your lids, you'll instantly create a new look.

KOHL TATOOS Who knew you were such a rebel ... Reserved for very special occasions.

What you'll need
- essential body oil
- body paint
- glitter
- a whole lot of imagination!

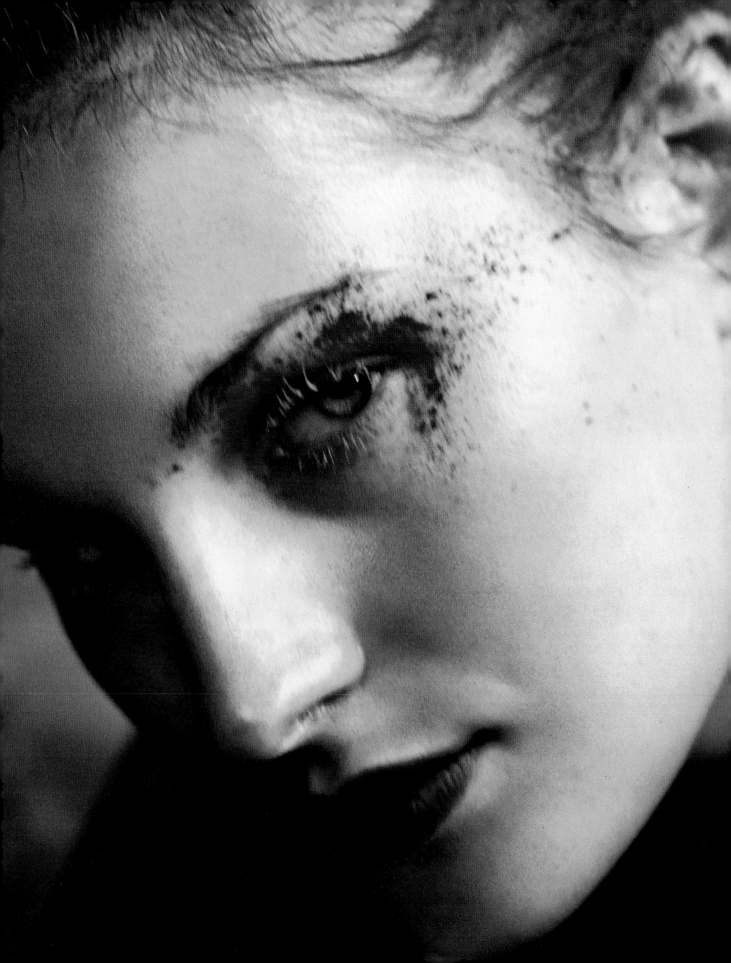

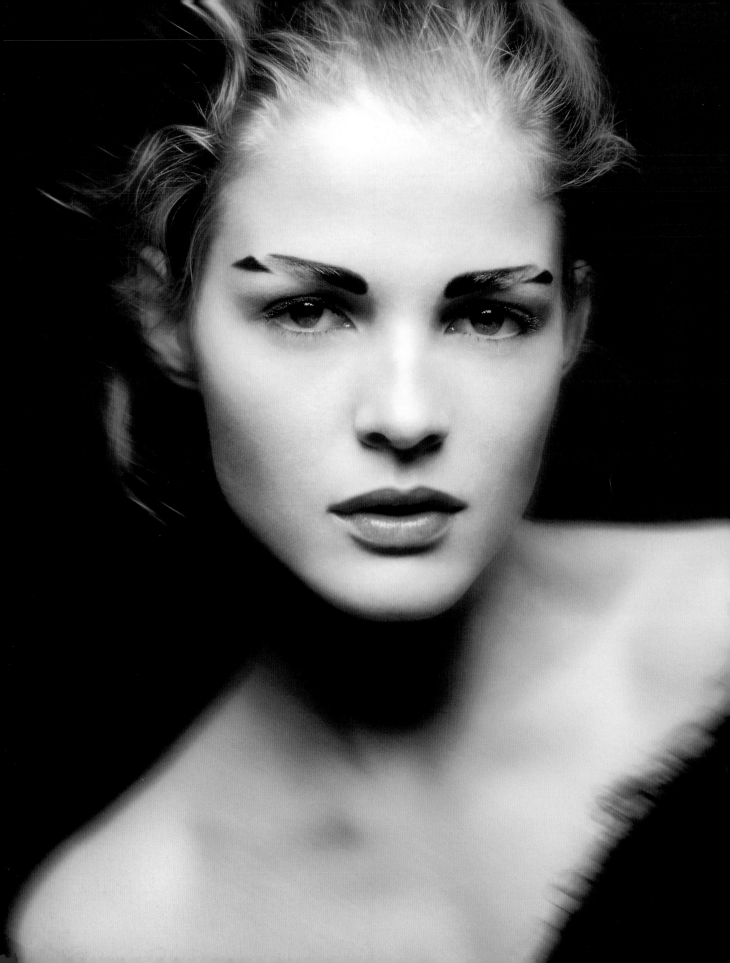

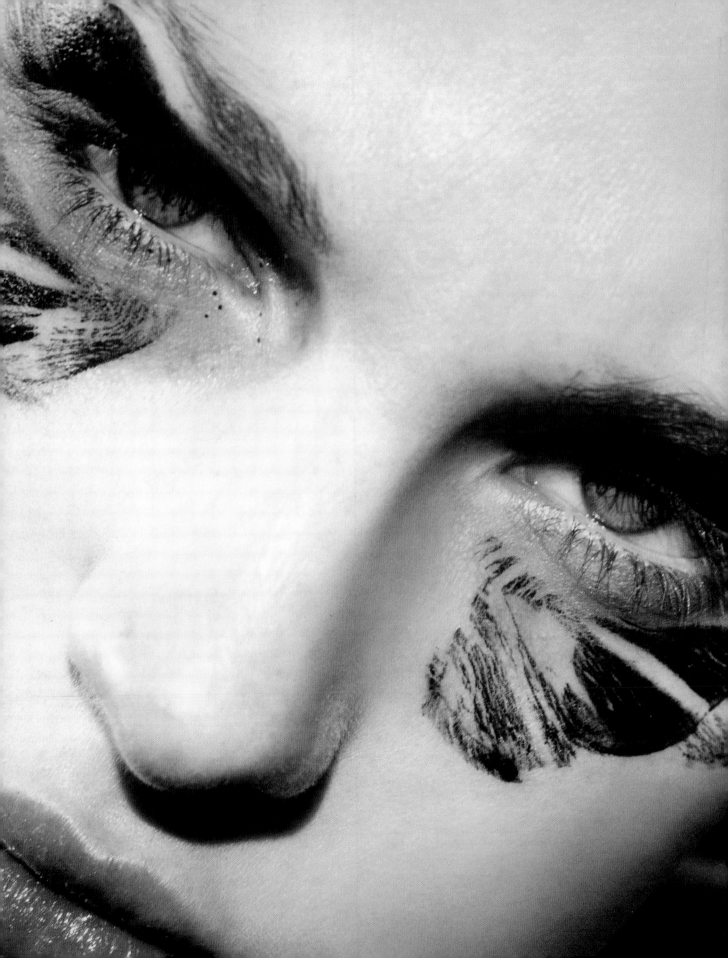

Credits

MAKEUP by **marie claire**

Production Editor: Thierry Lamarre
Author and Editorial Director: Josette Milgram
English Translation: Christopher Bouchard with Melanie Molnar
Creative Director and Layout Designer: Valérie Paturel
Copy Editor: Julie Bavant
Editorial Assistant: Adeline Lobut
Art Department: Domitille Peyron, Sylvie Creusy, Isabelle Teboul

First published in French by
Editons MARIE CLAIRE in 2006(c) 2006,
Editions Marie Claire - Société d'Information et de Créations (SIC)

This edition
Published in 2007 by Murdoch Books Pty Limited
www.murdochbooks.com.au

Murdoch Books Australia
Pier 8/9 23 Hickson Road
Millers Point NSW 2000
Phone: +61 (0) 2 8220 2000
Fax: +61 (0) 2 8220 2558

Murdoch Books UK Limited
Erico House, 6th Floor
93–99 Upper Richmond Road
Putney, London SW15 2TG
Phone: +44 (0) 20 8785 5995
Fax: +44 (0) 20 8785 5985

Project Manager: Anastasia McCall Hammond
Production: Monique Layt

The National Library of Australia Cataloguing-in-Publication Data:

Milgram, Josette.
Marie Claire makeup.
ISBN 9781741960150 (pbk.).
1. Beauty, Personal. 2. Cosmetics. I. Title.
646.7042

Printed by 1010 Printing International Limited, China in 2007.
PRINTED IN CHINA. Reprinted 2009, 2010.